Widow's Survival Guide

by Martin E. Levine, ChFC, CPA

Library of Congress Cataloging-In-Publication Data
Levine, Martin, 1953—
Widow's Survival Guide: The book you wish you didn't need...but you do.

Martin Levine—2nd ed.
TXU 863-776
ISBN 978-0-9669921-1-3

E-mail: mlevine@4TFG.com
www.4TFG.com

This book has been prepared especially to direct attention to problems which may arise in the event of death, and to provide answers to the questions most frequently asked.

IRS CIRCULAR 230 DISCLOSURE: To the extent that tax advise is contained in this workbook, such tax advise cannot be used by you, or any party to whom this workbook is shown, for the purpose of (i) avoiding penalties under the Internal Revenue Code or (ii) promoting, marketing or recommending the tax advice addressed herein to any other party.

Details of U.S. Government funded benefits, such as Social Security, Income Tax and Veterans' benefits may be subject to change with ongoing legislation. Always consult the proper authorities to determine the most current regulations and available benefits.

Links to other sites are for your convenience in locating related information and services. I and/or my agency do not maintain these other sites and have no control over the organizations that maintain the sites or the information, products or services these organizations provide. Although I or my agency, believe that the information from these organizations is reliable, we cannot guarantee its completeness or suitability for any purpose. Accordingly, I or my agency expressly disclaim any responsibility for the content, the accuracy of the information or the quality of products or services provided by the organization that maintains these sites.

DEDICATIONS

To my mother, Sylvia Levine

Widowed in 1972 at the age of 48

Like too many other women,
she was much too young to become a widow.

It was never easy. Her strength and love were there at a most painful time. She assured my brother Fred and myself that we were a team. All our decisions and choices were made for the team. It is still so today. In this spirit, with great love and pride I dedicate this book to my mother.

To Allison and Alexandra

For your love, support, and patience extended to me while writing this book.

ACKNOWLEDGMENTS

The writing of this book would not have been possible without the help of a few very special people.

First of all, the motivation to get up early and finally finish this book goes back to many evenings with a group of individuals taking a course with a company called Workability. Harlan, Lynette, Ann, Howard, Wendy, Susan, Maryann, and especially Ken, our group leader, created an atmosphere to help me realize, that I really wanted to write this book and that I could make this dream a reality.

The actual project got it's "second wind" from Dr. Marcia Posner. Her input was greatly appreciated and inspirational. Marcia, your humorous comments really did make me laugh. I knew after you reviewed my manuscript that I really had something special to offer.

For legal advice, my friend, Michael Donnelly, Esq., was always willing to review and clarify legal issues.

Like a lot of other areas in my life, when it came to testing my faith and commitment to "hang in there," I turned to a Rabbi, Rabbi Jeremy Widerhorn, to put the final touches on this dream.

I hope you enjoy it.

MEL

FOREWORD

It was my first time attending services to say kaddish, the Jewish prayer for the dead, since my husband Lou had died. Naturally, everyone was solicitous, but one young man went beyond the usual expressions of consolation. He invited me to call him anytime I needed help.

"What kind of help?" I asked, "like changing light bulbs?"

"I do that too," he smiled, "but I meant if you need help in figuring out financial records, that kind of thing. I remember how nervous my mother was after my dad died. She didn't know where to begin, but luckily my brother and I are accountants and we helped her. In fact, after so many of her friends asked for our help, over the years I put together a kind of 'widow's guide to financial peace and security.' I'll put it in your mailbox, if you want."

"Thanks," I replied. Truthfully, I was still too much in shock to begin to contemplate my finances and anyway, I was avoiding it as much as possible. My husband always took care of money matters and I never wanted to learn, despite his offers to teach me. He did numbers and business; I did books and writing. The only thing I knew about money was how to spend it.

A few days later, I found Marty's guide in my mailbox, hand delivered. I removed it and stuck it in a drawer. The first month I paid all bills with money in our joint checkbook account. If something needed my husband's name, I just signed it! After depleting the checkbook, I started hunting for bank passbooks. That's how people got money, I knew. They must be somewhere. I also knew that I could draw money from my husband's business, but no one had said anything to me about it. They were all waiting for me to give an indication of readiness to talk about finances, but I had a classic case of widow's denial. I also did not want them to find out how dumb I really was about money, when they all thought I was one smart lady!

In desperation, I dug out Marty's guide — and its first sentence calmed me down. By the second paragraph I knew that I could learn to do this. And thus began the journey of the first year of widowhood, following the guide, calling Marty when I needed to know something not in the guide, and using his advice and suggestions, even about consulting an estate lawyer as part of my "financial team." Eventually, I began to feel confident, making choices, making sense out of my new independent life. Not only did Marty teach me about the basics of bank practices, social security, investments and choosing a health plan, but also how to make lists and what kind of lists to make; how to judge my financial needs through these lists; how to deal with a business settlement, with children's and grandchildren's needs, but most of all — how to be able to form my own financial philosophy. When my husband was alive, we lived by his philosophy and it served us well, but now I was alone, the children grown. Did his philosophy still make sense at my age? What did I want out of the rest of my life? Marty's advice freed me to be my own person and to enjoy the years that are left.

Unknown to me, all along, Marty was working on a book to help widows like his mom, her friends, and now me. My questions and our discussions were being incorporated into the material he already had but was constantly revising. Finally, he gave me the manuscript to read. It was a jewel. I asked for a copy and it has become my blueprint for financial order and mental peace. I feel in control. Do yourself a favor. Don't stow this book on your bookshelf. Put it on your night table and read a chapter each night, not just when you need specific advice. It will not only help to maintain your solvency, but will also help you to establish priorities that will set you free.

Marcia W. Posner, MLS, PhD

TABLE OF CONTENTS

PART I - YOUR FIRST YEAR OF WIDOWHOOD

CHAPTER 1

CHAPTER 2

CHAPTER 3

CHAPTER 4

CHAPTER 5

CHAPTER 6

CHAPTER 7

CHAPTER 8

CHAPTER 9

CHAPTER 10

CHAPTER 11

PROLOGUE

It all began while preparing income tax returns, during the beginning of my adult working life, with one of the most creative accounting firms in New York City. In doing tax planning for clients, the questions asked would always go beyond the scope of the preparation of the tax return. For example, two of the more common questions were: will I be able to retire and should I make a contribution to a retirement plan? In hindsight, I know that these were good questions, since many years later, the same questions are still being asked. Although I no longer personally prepare tax returns, the questions are posed to me in my financial advisory practice if the client is concerned about retirement.

The phrase "money is near and dear to people" was true then and is still true today. In essence, I was in the business of helping my clients alleviate their fears about money and to reassure them that they were financially secure. Being there for my clients with timely advice was most rewarding. It was a role that suited my personality and coincided with the financial planning boom of the 1980's.

It was not until my father died, however, and my mother, brother and I had to sort out her financial choices, that I realized that my training was more and more perfect for a role as a financial advisor to widows. I could empathize with clients, particularly women like my mother, because I knew what they were going through. There was no one more qualified for the role. Along with my academic credentials: Masters of Business

Administration (MBA), Certified Public Accountant (CPA) and Chartered Financial Consultant (ChFC) degrees, I had something that was even more valuable, experience at being an advisor to a widowed mother.

I began to find a niche advising widows and they began finding me. This is when I realized that it was my duty to write this guide book for widows. After all, how many women have a Chartered Financial Consultant as a son?

CHAPTER 1

Play the Hand You Were Dealt

"Write the book, Marty," my mother said.

I wasn't certain. Although a great deal of my professional life has been spent advising people how to best organize — and maximize — their finances, I still hesitated.

My mother came over to me as I sat in the chair my father had sat in all those years ago. She rested her hand on my shoulder. Remember how it was when your father died?"

I looked up at her. And I smiled. I could smile and laugh now. I couldn't then. Not only had the unimaginable actually happened — I had lost my father and my mother had lost her husband after only 24 years of marriage. We quickly discovered that the world has little patience for sadness and grief.

It took two years before my mother was able to bring herself to go through my father's closet and give his clothes to charity. I remember that she cried then, drawing a suit jacket close to her face and saying, "I can still smell him in it."

Even now, there are moments of profound sadness. After my daughter was born, my mother would hold her and shake her head. "Your father would have adored her..."

"No one wants to be a widow," my mother said, her hand still on my shoulder. She shook her head sadly and her gaze turned to the window. "You spend your time and energy being a wife and mother for all those years..." Few women in my mother's generation gave much thought to money matters. Most women relied on their husbands to take care of the finances.

"No," she concluded, "not many of us were prepared to face that chapter in our lives."

I reached up and squeezed her hand. "What was it that Aunt Adele always said?" I asked.

She smiled. "You mean when you'd ask her how she managed?"

I nodded. My Aunt Adele is a lovely, woman who was a widow in her 30's with two small children.

She said, "I managed because I had to. I played the hand I was dealt. Did I have a choice?"

I smiled. I smiled hearing my mother capture the exact tone and inflection in my aunt's voice but I also smiled hearing the analogy. My mother and her sisters are great card players. As far back as I could remember, they would be in the kitchen at any family get-together, dealing a deck of cards, talking and laughing.

In hindsight, I wonder if they were subconsciously preparing themselves for the card game they would be forced to play later in their lives, when they were dealt a cruel hand -- when they would be left alone.

It was remarkable for me to learn many years later that part of the Old English definition of widow is an "extra hand at the card table." Unfortunately, that is sometimes how people, even friends, will regard you once you are no longer part of a couple. Some of the wives even get jealous that you'll go after their husband.

My mother patted my shoulder. "It takes time," she said quietly. "It takes time."

We all need time to address our grief.

Unfortunately, while our grieving continues in various ways throughout our lives, the demands of the world become pressing.

Over the years, I have taken special care to provide financial advice to women who have become widows. Having seen my mother go through that difficult transition, I want to make it easier for others. The Widow's Survival Guide provides the answers to the many questions most widows are too fearful to ask in public.

Summary — Chapter 1

1. Use markers (highlighters) to underline areas that are relevant to your situation.

HELPFUL WEBSITES:

www.aarp.org/families/grief_loss

CHAPTER 2

When and How to Take that First Step

"Beginnings are not easy," my mother said, "but so is knowing when to begin."

It does take time.

You have experienced a terrible loss. You will feel your loss emotionally and even physically. No one can tell you how long is the "right" amount of time to grieve. You have to give yourself the time you need to begin to adjust to your loss.

You will feel pressured to "get on with your life" from many different sources. You have to move forward at a pace that is comfortable for you. Take a deep breath before dealing with the demands of the world.

There are bills to pay and obligations to fulfill. No one can make sound financial decisions when they are in a state of emotional upheaval.

The decisions that you will be forced to confront will have a real impact on your future and the future of your family. They deserve the best consideration you can give them.

This is how this book, with a step by step approach, can help you face the demands ahead, for it is important to secure your future needs.

Begin when you are ready. While that answer might sound a little too clever (or maybe like no answer at all) it is the best possible answer. No one can tell you when you are ready. Only you can know that.

Don't be rushed into dealing with things before you are ready. If you do, your emotions will often get in the way. A lovely woman came to my office not long ago. She introduced herself to me, explaining that she had lost her husband just three months earlier.

"It's really horrible," she said, "starting over at sixty-seven."

"You're not really starting over," I explained, "You still have a great deal that you shared with your husband."

"Oh, I know, I know. It's just so strange. As much as I want to hold on to what we had — I also want to move on from it. Am I wrong to feel like that?" she asked.

"I don't think there is a right or wrong way to feel. Working through loss is a difficult process..." I said.

She nodded, took a deep breath and looked directly at me. "A month after Lenny died, I sold the vacation condominium we had purchased together. I couldn't imagine going there again ...without him. I think I got a fair price for it."

Although she did, in fact, receive a reasonable price for the condominium, she had acted in haste, letting her emotions dictate what should have been a more thoroughly considered financial decision. Sitting in my office, she expressed her ambivalence about not having the condo.

"I think it would have been a nice thing for my children to have..."

"Why do you think you sold it so soon after..?" I asked.

"I was just in one of those very down periods. It had been so sudden. Lenny hadn't been sick." She looked at me. "Heart attack." She sighed deeply. "I was looking through the photograph album and there were all these pictures of us..." She stopped and began to cry softly. "I'm sorry," she apologized. "I've told myself I wouldn't act like this — at least not in public. I couldn't imagine going back without him. I didn't want to be saddled with payments and upkeep...it just seemed that it would be an unnecessary burden and that it would remind me too much of Lenny. I knew I had to start making decisions. A friend of mine who had been widowed several years ago warned me about waiting too long to take control of my life. I figured I should just get started..."

As much as I sympathized with her, I could not help but think that she was a perfect example of "taking that first step" too soon. Although her desire not to be burdened with mortgage payments on a vacation home was a reasonable one, her decision to sell the condo was one she should not have made right away. Her timing was blurred by her emotions. She was "in a hurry" to do something and selling the condominium seemed like the right thing to do.

It might very well have been the case that selling the property was the wise, long-term decision. However, her decision to make the short-term gain — both financial and emotional — resulted in a fair financial gain which was not the best financial gain and perhaps not the right emotional (or personal) one as well. Being surrounded by family in a vacation setting can be very comforting, and she was already feeling ambivalent about the sale.

"Never rush an important decision."

Often, a death will result in a dramatic change in short-term finances, either through an insurance policy settlement or the proceeds of a retirement plan like an Individual Retirement Account (IRA) or pension.

Having the availability of such assets presents the opportunity to make a purchase or to make an investment. Clearly, no significant purchase or investment should be made in haste. Be cautious but don't become paralyzed by uncertainty.

Unfortunately, this difficult transition in your life is a balancing act and may be uncomfortable. Go slowly, planning is important in all financial decisions.

Take the time to understand as much as you can at first. That understanding will pay tremendous dividends in the future. Then go forward in measured, appropriate steps.

Learn to trust yourself.

However, listening to your own advice all the time can be dangerous.

Find someone to help you plan.

Planning is the key. If you "fail to plan, you plan to fail". So be open to new planning ideas. You will find yourself well on the road to gaining control over your life and your finances.

I recently went to a Jewish house of mourning during the "shiva" period (the seven days after burial), during which time the widow said with a gleam in her eye, "I can't believe I was able to take care of all the finances after Harry died and when he was sick!" You too have to believe in yourself and, believe you can take care of the finances!

Summary — Chapter 2

1. Begin when you are ready.
2. Never rush an important decision.
3. Learn to trust yourself.
4. Find someone to help you plan.
5. Remember, you can do it!

CHAPTER 3

Contact Social Security

"Be patient, but be persistent,"
my mother would say.

When Mona first came to me for financial advice, she had been collecting her husband's social security checks. I advised her that she needed to contact Social Security immediately and advise them that her husband had died. It is illegal to collect someone else's checks even if you believe that you are entitled to them.

Needless to say, that came as quite a shock to Mona.

"I thought I was entitled to continue to receive his benefits," she explained.

In Mona's case, she wasn't entitled because she was under fifty-nine and had no dependent children. Depending on your age, you may or may not be eligible to continue to receive your husband's benefits. You must notify Social Security when your husband passes away. If you continue to receive checks, do not cash them until you check that they're the right amount. The "rule of thumb" is if your husband was receiving benefits, you will be entitled to a reduced benefit or yours, whichever is greater.

If your husband wasn't receiving benefits, you may still be eligible to begin receiving his benefits.

In order to obtain an estimate of what your Social Security benefits will be, contact the Social Security Administration at 1-800-772-1213. Remember, the amount you will receive depends on what earnings your husband had during his working years. In addition, a modest death benefit may also be available to you.

While eligibility and benefit amounts are published annually, the Social Security system is difficult. Very few people — including many professionals — truly understand the workings of the system. My best advice to you is to refrain from trying to figure it out yourself. Contact your local Social Security office and try and determine where you stand and what benefits you are entitled to.

Be patient! There are few bureaucracies that can rival the Social Security Administration. Every delay that has been attributed to a bureaucracy has been attributed to the Social Security Administration — with just cause! Even when everything goes smoothly it may take a few weeks before receiving your benefits. (As of this writing, the Social Security has been improving on it's service.)

Your accountant or financial advisor should be able to help you determine if you are receiving the correct amount.

In addition to benefits for which you are eligible, your children may be eligible for individual benefits. If they are going to elementary or secondary school — or are disabled, there is a strong possibility that benefits are available to them.

Contact Social Security or your financial advisor as soon as possible to find out. When you go to social security, remember to bring the following:

- Your husband's social security number
- Your social security number
- Your children's social security numbers

- Your children's birth certificates
- Your marriage certificate
- Your husband's earnings statement for the current year
- Your husband's death certificate

If you are 70 years old, there is no advantage to waiting any longer to take your Social Security benefits (even if they are subject to income taxes).

Summary - Chapter 3

1. Do not cash your husband's checks — you may not be entitled to them!
2. Be patient, but be persistent.
3. Remember to bring your records when you go to Social Security.
4. Check with your advisor that the amount is correct.

HELPFUL WEBSITES:

www.ssa.gov

CHAPTER 4

Uncovering Your Husband's Financial Records

"Tell them not to panic," my mother told me. "I know it's hard to imagine but everything does work out."

Once the overwhelming shock of your loss begins to ease, you must slowly begin to sort out where you are. I mean that personally not just financially. Hopefully, your basic needs of food, shelter, and clothing are not at risk.

The best place to take stock of "where you are" is to take a look at where your husband made his living and what stage of life he was in.

What Did Your Husband Do For A Living?

Sole Proprietor - Being in Business or Practice for Yourself

One of my clients was widowed by a man who had been in business for himself but who did not plan for the eventuality of his death.

This problem is very common amongst sole proprietors. Once they die, the business dies with them. The only thing that is commonly left is the real estate, materials, tools, and office equipment.

"Because of the nature of Joe's business, he was the business. When he died, the business died with him. The only thing of value was the real estate itself." She shook her head sadly. "If only he would have thought to have taken out a life insurance policy as a business owner."

What was true of this client's husband is also true of most licensed professionals — lawyers, doctors, engineers or accountants. Unless one of your children is able to step in and continue your husband's practice in that profession, his practice will have to be sold.

Closing the business or practice

Accounts and notes receivables should be collected. Final accounts payable and outstanding expenses should be paid. Remaining cash should be taken.

In certain professions, such as accounting, the clientele is saleable. Additionally, if your husband had been at the same location for a long time and had established goodwill, then his practice might be worth more.

Your husband's accountant can help with the final accounting and with completing any unfinished business. Your lawyer should also be involved in the final stages of your husband's business to make sure you do not have any on-going liabilities.

Employee

While your situation might be simplified if your husband was an employee, you may be entitled to other benefits. These include group life insurance, accidental death insurance, pension or profit sharing plans and financial planning.

You should contact the human resource or benefits department in matters of life insurance and benefits. In all likelihood, the only document you will need in order to receive benefits will be an official, signed death certificate.

You should ask for a copy of the pension or profit sharing plan. Once you have received this, you should consult with your financial advisor or your accountant to determine which option is best for you and your situation. How you receive these benefits could affect your own retirement.

Choices can be made after your benefits are clarified and a complete strategy can be developed based on your needs.

More and more, large companies are providing financial planning services for family members of deceased employees. In these cases, the employer will contact you to offer these services. If you choose to take advantage of this offer, the outside financial planning company is contacted by the employer and then a counselor contacts you for an appointment date.

Retired

If, at the time of his death, your husband was retired from a business or company, you might still be entitled to some benefits. For example, some employer retirement plans allow retirement monies to stay and be reinvested even though the employee is no longer employed. Other pension plans will continue paying you the same benefit, a reduced benefit, or sometimes, no further benefit.

Other companies have plans which, in addition to pension and profit sharing plans, call for non-qualified deferred compensation payments. These plans have monies left with the company which are yours based on a written agreement.

Regardless of your husband's employment status at the time of his death, you would be well advised to speak with your chosen financial counselor in order to receive all benefits you are entitled to. In addition, you want to be sure to receive those benefits in a way that minimizes your tax burden and maximizes your financial well-being.

The various pension, retirement, and non-qualified deferred compensation plans seem to conspire to make up an "alphabet soup" of legalize. Each kind of plan has certain benefits and certain pitfalls. *Options must be laid out for you so that your financial health is secure.*

You will want to see the various "income tax projections" for each option; and the "cash flow projection," which projects *how much money you will have available now and later on.*

With some of the previously mentioned items uncovered, you will be in a better position to understand the financial position in which you've been left. Depending on the particulars of your situation and the knowledge you bring into the process, this can be a very simple step or one that seems too overwhelming to even contemplate.

After you've gone through his business and employment records, you need to make sure to account for all his life insurance.

Life Insurance

"I knew he had several life insurance policies and some through the business. I knew about them. But, I couldn't find them when I needed them."

Finding documents is often a frustrating challenge during this time. Life insurance policies are important but don't let yourself get overly stressed if you cannot locate them.

Papers tend to show up again. Within one year something will come in the mail that may be needed. If you cannot find the original document, it is possible to receive duplicate statements and replacement policies.

Life insurance companies can provide you with a lost

policy form which can be used instead of the original policy. A return of the original policy along with the death claim form and death certificate is normally all that is required by the insurance company before a death claim is paid to you.

Remember to get extra death certificates from the funeral director for your future use.

The most important thing is — don't panic! Things will work out. Remember we all have different organizational skills and methods. Even someone who has an impeccable filing system at work might have something far more informal at home. And even someone with a great home filing system can misplace things!

Life insurance policies can be traced. Contact the broker or agent who handles your insurance policies. If you do not have an agent or if you're not sure if there were any life insurance policies, check for canceled bills or go through twelve months of canceled checks.

It is a good idea to contact your husband's place of business to find out what policies were held for him at work.

If your husband put his life insurance policy or policies in a trust, it may likely be an irrevocable trust. An irrevocable trust's main purposes is to keep the insurance proceeds out of his estate and your estate, creditor protection and keep the proceeds in the family. You still have access to the money, but after you die, just as when your husband died, the proceeds are not subject to possible estate taxes. You'll need to open a trust checking account, if one is not already opened, and help decide where you are going to invest the money if you are a co-trustee. (There are a few small rules which you will have to follow but your financial advisor or attorney should be able to make these very clear to you.)

However, I can not emphasize enough that you should not get unduly nervous or worried if things don't turn up readily. As I mentioned before, lost policy forms, duplicate statements and replacement policies can — and will — be ordered and sent to you.

One of the papers that your search will hopefully turn up will be the original of your husband's Will. If you cannot locate his Will at home or at his work, check either with the attorney who drafted it or at the bank safe deposit box.

Safe Deposit Boxes

There are a great many reasons to have safe deposit boxes. Sometimes they pose obstacles and hurdles after the death of a loved one. If you and your husband had a safe deposit box, you, as a joint lessee on the account, are only allowed to enter the box and make copies of any papers expressing your husband's wishes concerning burial, deed to a cemetery plot or proof of membership in a burial society. The original papers must be returned to the box and the box sealed until a release is obtained from the State Tax Department.

If, however, the safe deposit box is in your husband's name alone, you will have a very difficult time getting into it. Once the bank has been notified that your husband has passed away, it will seal the safe deposit box until a release from the State Tax Department is presented.

You might want to use this knowledge about safe deposit boxes to insure that your loved ones do not have a similar difficulty when you pass away. Have another family member get a safe deposit box in their name.

Do not keep your Will or funeral documents in your safe deposit box!

If you are not sure if you have a safe deposit box, you will be able to look for a charge in one of the following places in an effort to locate one: past bank statements, a previously paid bill, or incoming bill through the mail.

There are a number of alternatives for storing your important papers.

You should, of course, purchase a fireproof box, safe, or filing cabinet for your home. Make sure someone else has the key or combination as well as the location of the safe. In this way, you bypass any need to deal with a bank or other institution.

Move forward slowly. There will be some people who will infuriate you and others who you will swear are angels sent from heaven to aid you. Focus on the angels.

Chapter 4 — Summary

1. Check your husband's current or former place of employment for financial records. Do not get overly stressed if you cannot locate papers. They will turn up or be replaced.
2. Options must be laid out for you so that your financial health is secure (cash flow and income tax projections).
3. Understand the financial position in which you've been left.
4. Ideally, you want to enlist the help of family if available, but more likely a financial advisor.

CHAPTER 5

When Your Husband Dies Without a Will

"It was a good thing we had just updated our Wills before Daddy died," my mom exclaimed.

Even if your husband did not have a Will, the good news is that your state government has one for you. Unfortunately, that is the bad news as well. Dying without a Will will cost more money and create delays in the disbursement of his estate. Not having a Will when one dies is called "dying intestate". There are certain rules which dictate who gets the assets that are in his name alone. For example, in addition to yourself, your child may receive part of the assets directly. There is also something else to be aware of — if a child is under 18 years old at his father's death, a court appointed guardian will be required to manage your child's share. The court will probably appoint you as the guardian, but a bond may have to be posted along with annual accountings of income and expenses. There are also limits on how to invest the child's money. Hopefully, the guardianship will not last a long time and this hindrance will become a bad memory.

Seek out an attorney who has worked with estates where no Will was left. The best way to find a "trust and estate lawyer" is through a recommendation. Ask a friend, family member, or existing advisor who they would recommend. If you cannot come up with anybody, you can always look for seminars given by attorneys and financial planners. They are usually advertised in the local newspaper and are generally very informative. Some of the attorneys who speak are actually very good.

Ask beforehand what their hourly rate is. Do not hire an attorney who charges a percentage of the estate value.

If the estate is simple, an attorney will have a good idea of what the fee will be. A complicated estate however will be a little more difficult to determine and can get very expensive. The estimated fee usually does not include additional charges incurred if the estate gets audited by the Internal Revenue Service.

Interview more then one attorney. See which one you like and if their fees are comparable. Fees begin at $200 per hour and up. Handling simple estates can begin at $1,000. Additional court costs may be required.

Chapter 5 — Summary

1. Your financial future can be affected if your husband died without a Will.
2. A carefully planned document could have simplified your future. Don't make the same mistake twice.
3. Seek legal help!

CHAPTER 6

Getting Organized

"For a long time, I didn't throw out a thing. Not a receipt, not a bill, not an invoice," my mother said.

When you are ready to take the first steps to get yourself organized, you will have to take stock of yourself and your financial situation. This is the same as taking an "inventory of your stock" if you were in business. (See Figure 1 in this chapter.)

Make Lists!

Most of us are familiar with the advantage of writing lists. My wife wallpapers the refrigerator door with dates and things to be done.

Ideas

You may get an idea for making money — a potential business idea which should be written down to discuss with someone later on. Some great and valuable ideas have been written on the backs of cocktail napkins. Never short change yourself. Give yourself a chance. Some of the greatest success stories in life have come out of second or third careers. Don't take writing things down too lightly, particularly when they are easy to forget.

You may see advertisements in the newspaper making claims on specific rates of return for your money. Make a list of what bank or mutual fund company it is and what return on your money is being promised. This way when you meet with your investment advisor, you will be able to go over the list and see how that compares with what he or she is offering you.

Benefits of Retaining Lists

The benefits of records and lists cannot be underestimated. They help you locate and identify assets and expenses. Once items are listed, they are easily accessible for evaluating how your investments are doing (see Figures 2 - 6 in this chapter).

An additional benefit of all these lists, beyond their immediate usefulness to your financial status and state of mind, is the amount of time you will be saving your heirs. These lists that follow, will save your heirs the trouble and uncertainty of identifying what you owned when you pass away. (I will discuss this further with you in Part II "Planning For Your Future" on the benefit of lists for your own estate planning.)

You are going through quite a lot during the first year. You are really in a state of shock. What you think as — "Look, I'm O.K., look how well I am doing!" is shock, denial and adrenaline. Because of this - thoughts go in and out of your mind like skittish butterflies. Lists, therefore are the path to *sanity!*

Lists

Figures 1-7

List 1 - General Inventory - List of all relevant financial information

List 2 - Financial Obligations (Liabilities)

List 3 - Monthly Expenses

List 4 - Possible Quarterly, Semi-Annual, and Annual Expenses

List 5 - Income Sources

List 6 - Assets

List 7 - Gift List

List 1

Pre-List (General Inventory)

List of all relevant financial information

- Bank accounts-joint, individual, in trust
- Life insurance policies-your husband's and yours-group and personal
- Retirement plans-your husband's and yours
- Real estate
- Brokerage accounts
- Mutual funds
- Business interests-partnership & corporation

Figure 1

List 2
List of Financial Obligations* (Liabilities)
as of (date)

Item	Owed To	Outstanding Balance	Date Finished	Monthly Payment
Mortgage-1				
Mortgage-2				
Equity loan				
Auto lease				
Auto loan				
Personal loan				
1 Credit card				
2 Credit card				
3 Credit card				
4 Credit card				
5 Credit card				
Gas card				
Gas card				
Other				
Totals				

*Financial obligations are IOUs with balances that you are paying off over time. These are part of your monthly expenses.

Figure 2

List 3

Monthly Expenses

Cash withdrawals

Financial obligations

(monthly payments-List 2)

Rent

Mortgage

Maintenance

Electric, gas & oil

Telephone

Health insurance

Cable TV

Bottled water

Trash pickup

Landscaping maintenance

Food

Clothing

Child care

Dry cleaning

Prescriptions

Monthly Expenses (continued)

Doctor visits ______

Dentist visits ______

Gas - auto ______

Auto - lease ______

Entertainment ______

Club dues ______

Hair & nails ______

Other miscellaneous ______

Total Monthly Expenses

Figure 3

List 4

Possible Quarterly, Semi-Annual or Annual Expenses
(One time expenses can also be listed here)

	Quarterly	Semi-Annual	Annual
Estimated income taxes			
Federal			
State			
Real estate taxes			
(School, town, village, etc.)			
Home insurance			
Water			
Heating fuel			
Repairs and maintenance			
Education - Tuition			
Insurance			
Medical			
Dental			
Home health care			
Nursing home			
Life insurance			
Disability			
Auto insurance			
Auto - maintenance			
Charity			
House of worship			

Possible Quarterly, Semi-Annual or Annual Expenses (continued) (One time expenses can also be listed here)

	Quarterly	Semi-Annual	Annual
Vacations			
Professional fees			
Tax preparation			
Financial consultant			
Other			

Totals (carry below)			
Total Monthly (from List 3)	________	x12=	________
Total Quarterly	________	x 4=	________
Total Semi-Annual	________	x 2=	________
Total Annual	________	x 1=	________
Total Expenses per Year			________

Figure 4

List 5

How much Income do you have coming in each month?

Potential Income Sources	
Social Security	
Pensions	
Earned income from work	
Salary	
Bonus	
Commissions	
Rental income	
Interest - Tax free	
Interest - Taxable	
Dividends	
Mutual funds	
Annuities	
Trusts (1)	
Trusts (2)	
Partnerships	
Business distribution	
Health insurance reimbursement	
Other	
Total Monthly Income	
Total Income other then monthly	
CDs	
Bonds	
Annual Income	

Figure 5

List 6

Assets

Cash in Bank

Money Market

Amounts owed you

  Mortgages

  Notes

Brokerage Accounts

Individual held stocks

Individual held bonds

Mutual funds

Annuities

Other investments

Retirement plans

 IRA|SEP

 Pension, Profit Sharing, Keogh

 Tax Deferred Annuities

Real Estate

  Home

  Vacation home

  Rental property

Life insurance policies

  Cash value (   )

  Death benefit

Personal property

  Art work

  Household effects

  Jewelry

Total

Figure 6

List 7

Gift List

To Whom	What Item	Location

Figure 7

The Check Book

If you are not sure how your husband kept the check book (or what creative methods he employed to keep it balanced) or even if managing the check book was a "team" effort, you might find it easier simply to start fresh and open a new checking account.

You might eventually have to establish a separate estate account. Consult with your accountant about the advisability of this in your situation. Once an estate is settled, which means that all bills have been paid and all assets have been distributed, no extra accounts need to be kept.

If you do decide to establish a new, personal checking account, your initial deposit could be the proceeds from your husband's life insurance policy. Many banks offer free checking if you maintain a minimum balance. This way, you can avoid bank charges.

There is no sound financial reason for beginning a new checking account. You might want to move the account to a more convenient location. Do not set up a new joint account with a child, unless you understand the risks associated with doing so. A child who is a signature on an account has the right to withdraw money from that account at any time without your say. The other potential problem is that you have lost some of your privacy.

Taking care of your financial commitments can sometimes become a social happening.

For example, whenever my mother is planning on making a trip to the bank she includes a number of other activities and chores. Shopping can become a social scene. Occasionally lunch with a friend and perhaps an art gallery visit. It is imperative to have a plan for leaving your house and to engage in outside entertainment.

There is no way to understand how important it is for you to involve yourself in activities that bring you into contact with people. Don't let your sad experience turn you into a shut-in. Do not be a prisoner in your own home.

If a trip to the bank is your best opportunity to do that then that's a reason in and of itself to involve yourself in your financial matters.

Banking is an extremely competitive business. Free checking. ATM cards and machines. Small considerations. Take advantage of what your bank can offer you. If you feel that you can do better — change banking institutions.

If you do avail yourself of an ATM machine, be sure to record each cash withdrawal in your checkbook.

I recommend that you do not use an ATM at night — especially if you are alone. You must remember safety when involving yourself with cash withdrawals.

Balancing the checkbook

First some checkbook terms:

Automatic deposits-transfers from a savings, money market account or credit line

Outstanding checks-have not yet cleared (been cashed) by the bank

Automatic payments - payments out of account

While many people suppose that there is some magic involved in balancing a checkbook, it really is nothing more than a question of adding and subtracting correctly. Remember, your bank statement might not reflect the checks you've actually written so you need to take that into account when reconciling your figures with the bank's figures.

Balancing your checkbook is an important task. It allows you to confirm the amount of money you have in your checkbook and it also allows you to question the bank when you think it is in error — and that does sometimes happen.

Your balanced checkbook is your best documentation for avoiding overdrafts and for discovering banking errors.

There is also a tremendous sense of accomplishment when you actually do balance the figures. This is evident by the many people who boast to me of managing to "balance" their checkbooks when their results are within five to ten dollars of what their bank statement reflects.

If you are like another one of my clients, Mary Beth, convinced that you will never, be able to balance your checkbook nor would you even enjoy attempting to do so, there are record-keeping or bookkeeper services available that provide this service to you at minimal cost. Your accountant might be able to help you with this as well.

Even if you are convinced that you will never be able to balance your checkbook, you might want to talk to someone at the bank who could show you what to do.

If all else fails, you want to be sure that you don't overdraw your account. Therefore, any measures you take to ensure that you always have more money in your account than you write checks against will be satisfactory. (Ask your bank if you qualify for an overdraft line of credit for extra protection.)

There is no worse feeling in the world than having a check "bounce," especially when you are trying to establish your own financial independence.

Some banks, when you've gotten to know them, will call you when you are overdrawn. This way, you can come in and make a deposit to cover the overdraft (even though they have already paid the check).

Another item you want to be aware of is uncollected funds. Uncollected funds are out of state deposits you make which take days to clear before checks can be drawn against them. If your average balances are high enough, some banks credit your deposits up to $2,500 - $5,000 immediately no matter where the deposited check is from.

One of the cruel realities of our society is that there are people who prey on the vulnerability of a new widow. You are considered "easy pickings." This is particularly true with investments. Buyer Beware! is a saying that too often falls on deaf ears for unknowing widows.

Don't let this turn into the truth!

If anyone claims that you or your late husband owes money, ask for proof. In this age of computers — and computer errors — there are times when someone honestly believes they are owed money. In fact, poor record keeping or a computer error will provide wrong information.

You do not owe anything until someone is able to properly demonstrate that you do. Insist on proof!

How Should All These Papers Be Organized?

An accountant's dream world is one in which everything is filed correctly and in which all columns are neat. That is, after all, an accountant's stock in trade. There is a good reason for this and it has to do with the realities with which they deal. I should know this since I was an accountant for almost ten years.

Being organized makes keeping track of important papers infinitely easier. And, if that important piece of paper is easily found, the decisions that have to be made based on the information it holds will be that much sounder.

Your kitchen may be neat and organized. Closets and drawers. You might be the very ideal of domestic organization. Your phone book and old PTA lists are still exactly where you want them to be. However, this may be the first time you've been confronted with the need to organize your "papers."

If this is the case, the prospects may seem daunting but they are really no more difficult than keeping track of birthdays, anniversaries, doctor appointments, or theater tickets.

My advice is to institute a filing system using either file folders or large envelopes. Some banks and investment companies have begun to send out statements already three-hole punched. If that is the case with your bank or investment, you might consider purchasing a binder to keep those papers organized.

Once you have your folders, you need to label them clearly. One folder that you need is your "HOUSE" folder.

Your "HOUSE" folder would hold all papers relevant to your house expenses. If you own a house or apartment, some of these expenses — capital improvements

— may be needed when and if you sell your property. Your financial advisor or accountant will counsel you regarding the exemptions and benefits which apply.

Other folders should hold your medical expenses, utilities, car, insurance, etc. A typical bill, such as tax notices (except for real estate taxes), should be reviewed by an accountant or tax attorney to determine their applicability. Your advisor can also help you decide whether these bills will be received regularly and need their own filing folder.

How to File

After you pay your typical monthly bills, mark "paid" with the amount, check number, and date on the statement portion. Then file the paid receipt in a labeled file.

Once you become comfortable with your filing system, you'll find that every aspect of your personal finances becomes simpler. It is also critical to have a desk set up in a place where you are comfortable working.

"I wouldn't believe that I could be so organized," Alice told me after putting all her papers in order. "But after I did, I felt so much more in control."

Being in control is exactly what you want to strive towards.

It's not only possible to be in control, but very achievable if you practice what I'm saying.

All organizational tasks seem daunting at first. Even if your husband was organized, you might be more comfortable with a different system, one more suited to your way of doing things. All that is important is that it works for you. Advisors can — and should adapt. Once you have things the way you want them, evaluating your financial decisions will be a good deal easier.

One file or folder that you should definitely include in your system is a file for your accountant or tax preparer. Call that file: "INCOME TAXES." Also put the year on the file in a visible place in case you ever have to go back to find something. While you may abhor this file, having it will simplify your life. Remember, you tax preparer will need your December investment statements (which you may not receive until February or March of the following year). Another good way of keeping track of potentially tax deductible items is to use a yellow highlighter in your checkbook register. This is particularly good when your only receipt is your canceled check.

You might prefer to go through each check when your bank statement comes in monthly and segregate the checks that you'll need later on for your accountant (see Figure 8).

The Recipe Box Technique

A box the size of a recipe box for "income tax" items will do with the tabs or categories divided as follows:

- taxes paid
- charities*
- medical
- professional fees
- educational expenses
- business\investment expenses

*Charities solicit all year long, so alphabetize the solicitations, throw out duplicates, and pay them all once a year. If you want to pay monthly or more often, alphabetize canceled checks in your income tax folder.

Figure 8

Husband's Estate. Utilities. Car Expenses. Medical. Mortgage payments. Insurance (life, health — Medicare and/or long-term care). Social Security. Credit cards. These are just some of the files you may want to create.

Your filing system will depend on your circumstances and needs.

Once you've established your filing system, you should update the files annually. (Not every file will be repeated every year.) The past year's papers should be put in storage — accessible but out of the way. You can use transfer files or a filing cabinet for both old and current files.

"I just can't stand the thought of having all these papers all over the place!"

Don't worry, I will explain below that you don't have to become a complete "pack rat" of paperwork. However, setting up a filing system is important for saving you time and aggravation. When you need to speak with your advisors, you will be prepared. When you prepare your income tax, your paperwork will be at your fingertips. Remember, a professional's time is worth money. The more time you spend organizing your own records, the less time the professional will need, and therefore, the more modest your bill will be.

Recently a new client of mine, Millie, indicated that the accountant used to come to her home and do her taxes. "We were spending more time on stories about the children then the taxes," she exclaimed. She finally realized that she was paying for his time and was better off just sending him the papers. The result was that the bill to prepare her tax return went down.

As I noted above, your filing system provides for other benefits as well. It establishes a good place for you to evaluate where you are financially. With an effective and efficient filing system, you, as a single women, will be able to determine how some of your expenses need to be updated, using Figures 3 & 4 in this chapter. Insurance is one prime example. I will discuss this further with you in Part II on "Planning For The Future."

Your filing system will also benefit your heirs when they are called upon to manage your estate and all your assets.

Throw Out Unnecessary Papers

My mother was right to have been cautious in the early part of her widowhood. As she became more comfortable with her role in her own financial status, however, she came to feel confident about which papers she needed to keep. I remember the row of bank statements which must have represented ten to fifteen years that was finally thrown out when she sold the house. I asked her years later why she kept all those statements and her answer went right to the heart of the matter. "I thought I needed them," she told me.

Another example of excess accumulation is investment papers such as mutual fund statements which contain the activity of the previous month. The first statement for the year shows January's activity. The next statement will show both January's activity as well as February's. If the figures for January match both documents, the first can be discarded.

This is true for each subsequent statement. The final statement for the year, received in December, is the only one which you need to keep for your records.

This same process holds true for most brokerage accounts. If you have any questions or doubts regarding what paperwork you need to keep, ask your financial advisor for guidance.

Old bills and records should be recycled where they could do some good instead of collecting dust in your filing system.

Keep Track of Important Dates

Some payments are due at regularly "irregular" intervals. While monthly payments are easier to keep track of, these other payments must be made on time. Estimated taxes, insurance payments, and other such "quarterly" or "semi-annual" payments should be noted on a yearly calendar.

In the case of estimated taxes, your accountant or tax preparer will provide you with the dates they are due when your income taxes are prepared. Remember to ask if you should pay your state estimated tax payment by December 31 in order for it to be deductible on your federal return. It is normally due on January 15 of the following year.

While you do not have to pay your estimated taxes on a quarterly basis (deciding instead to pay the entire tax burden on April 15th), you should be aware that the decision to put off these payments will result in an additional interest and penalty charge. The purpose of the estimated taxes is to allow the state and federal governments to generate a steady income rather than waiting for a very large windfall on April 15th.

Become comfortable with using a yearly calendar to mark important financial dates and deadlines. This practice will aid you in your cash flow planning. There are few things more unsettling then "surprises" at the end of the month.

"I was shocked when I learned how much I would have to pay in income taxes," one of my new clients, Betty, complained.

With some sound advice along with some simple bookkeeping and planning, you should be able to plan for those large payments so that the money is available when you need it — think ahead carefully and set aside money periodically. This will enable you to remit required payments without withdrawing large amounts of your capital.

How Long Should Important Papers Be Kept?

I am asked this question all the time. Clearly, the difficult part of the question is, what constitutes an "important paper?" When I ask my clients what they think are important papers, they inevitably answer with, "Income tax."

Personal income tax returns and related back-up documentation should be kept for three years. Business tax returns and related back-up should be kept for six years. ("Related back-up documentation" means the bills, canceled checks, invoices, etc. that support the numbers on the tax return.) Back-up documentation is kept in the event of an audit. Even if you got rid of most of this documentation, it could be duplicated if you need it. For example, copies of canceled checks can be ordered from the bank.

Once again, the underlining advice is, don't worry and don't panic.

If you find yourself in a situation you don't understand, ask for help. There are professional financial advisors who will be able to answer your questions on the phone or will tell you what papers to send them. You will feel good when these problems are solved.

Chapter 6 — Summary

1. You must take stock (inventory) of your financial position by using my lists in figures 1 - 6.
2. Make "to do" lists and get a good calendar to keep track of important dates.
3. Be comfortable with your bank location.
4. Get yourself set up with a desk and a filing system.
5. Be in control.
6. You are not only doing this for today, but also for the future.
7. Look into saving important papers by using a scanner.

CHAPTER 7

Your Husband's Business Agreements

"It's a good thing Daddy had sold the business at full value before he died, I never would have received the same value for his share," my mother told us.

A shareholder or partnership agreement can also simplify your future, if your husband had one or more co-shareholders or partners. These agreements can clearly state terms for disposal of your husband's business assets.

If there was no business agreement, then your husband's ownership interest would be transferred to you or your children according to the provisions of his Will.

While there are some exceptions, the optimal situation is transference of ownership interest to you and not your children. Then the choice can be yours to sell or keep the ownership and run the business.

Should you decide to continue the business, consult the key members and advisors of the firm. If you have no experience or if you are unfamiliar with the business, assuming such an important role is ripe with pitfalls. The remaining owners or key employees may not be pleased to be in business with their former partner's wife.

Your husband's business agreement may have a buyout clause that would allow your husband's partners to buy you out with life insurance or notes (IOUs). If there is no such clause, then it would be worthwhile for an accountant of your choosing to be brought in to review the situation and clearly explain to you your options.

A buy-out can be beneficial for you and your children. The money realized from the life insurance proceeds can also be used by the child active in the business to buy-out the interests of the child who is not active in the business. In this way, equalization is created among your family members.

Such a sense of fairness and equality will go a long, long way toward your own sense of happiness and well-being.

Too many times, the death of a parent results in hard feelings between children. This situation frays and often fragments families. A sound business agreement regarding children in the business can go a long way toward avoiding this terrible predicament. Consider it for yourself if your husband had no "business continuity" plan.

"If only we would have had it in writing," is a phrase I commonly hear. When a plan is not in writing, the chance for a successful transition can be much more difficult. It depends on the parties involved. This is a big reason why over 70% of family owned business's never make it to the next generation.

The following are two "real life" scenarios which demonstrate what can happen without a written plan:

There was a stepson, adopted by his mother's second husband, who wants to buy out the second husband from his own business - because the poor guy had a stroke! He's offering them too little and the man doesn't want to be bought out.

The other scenario involves a man and his partner (brother-in-law), where the partner has been helpless from a stroke for 10 years and has received his full draw for all that time!

The possible outcomes are endless. One possibility that you can insist on in writing is a lifetime income stream, based on the value of the business. A buyout can be tricky. If no agreement is in place, demand more, so you can have a better bargaining chip. Remember to cover for contingencies in case the nature of the business changes.

Get involved! Switch your attention from homemaking, hobbies, etc. - to what is going on <u>right now</u> in your husband's business.

Summary - Chapter 7

1. Taking over the business is ripe with pitfalls, particularly if you have no experience with it. Be careful!
2. Remember, your husband was probably given the advice on which "business continuity" agreement should be in place.
3. If no agreement was in place, seek professional advice on your best options.

CHAPTER 8

Learning Your Financial Worth/Standing

"I do not know if I would have been able to figure it out without the help of my sons," my mom would later say.

Even women who have worked most of their adult lives sometimes find this process troubling. Most of the time, your husband has been responsible for the financial planning and overall business management of your life.

"My earnings were slightly more than his during the last few years," Susan shared with me during our appointment. "But I still didn't have any idea about our finances. I didn't know until after he passed away, that he had made a number of investments. It was only later, when I had to know, that I learned the details of our finances."

Susan was in a position that is not that unusual these days. More and more women work out of the house, bringing in much needed income to the family's finances. However, some of these women remain completely in the dark about their finances even though they are contributing to the economy of the household.

In Susan's case, she was surprised by the number of investments her husband had made in mutual funds, retirement plans, a brownstone, and the particulars of the time-share that they owned for vacations. His decisions had been good ones. Their money had not been "frittered away." However, some of his investments required constant attention to keep them maximized.

For example, the brownstone had four rent-paying tenants. Collecting the rent was not the difficult part, but the maintenance did require attention. When Susan's husband was alive, he managed to take care of regular maintenance. Now that responsibility was Susan's alone.

Susan managed to relieve herself of the day-to-day headaches of maintaining her property by finding a management company to handle them for her. Her days were no longer interrupted by telephone calls from tenants. More importantly, she didn't feel the constant tension of anticipating those phone calls. Finding a management company is best done through referrals. Their fee of between 5% and 15% was worth it to her. If this is unavailable, the next best thing is to ask one of your current advisors who they might recommend.

Of course, Susan was still responsible for the cost of repairs, but fortunately, her husband had invested in a profitable property and she benefited by his real estate investment.

Things were not so simple for Betty. Her husband had used the "scraps of paper and old envelopes" method of business dealings. His method was capricious and completely without organization. He kept track of their finances in a code that only he could break.

"It was most confusing," Betty said, the exasperation still evident in her voice months later. "All those pieces of paper were like a jig saw puzzle."

"I remember once I went with him to the accountant to do our taxes and he brought out all these envelopes. The accountant was most annoyed, but with my husband there to explain everything, things worked out."

"Once he was gone..." She shook her head. "We couldn't make heads or tails of these notations."

"To make matters worse, there were papers I didn't find until two to three months later. Tucked away in file boxes and folders in his office and at home."

"It was a nightmare."

It took Betty much longer than that to sort out simple things and understand what money was coming in and going out. Canceled checks were made payable to cash and it was difficult to know what the money was used for.

For Betty, getting herself organized demanded consultation with a financial consultant. Without one, she would have been totally confused. She happily discovered that she was financially sound.

"I don't know if I ever would have figured it out without help," she shook her head in amazement. "I did not know we were getting income from an investment he had made during our fifth year of marriage!"

Both Betty and Susan confronted the same need — to understand the position in which they were left. That task was made more or less difficult depending on their ability to get a grip on their finances and getting someone to help them with the management responsibilities.

The important thing to remember is that you cannot become frustrated. If your husband was not an organized person, the likelihood is that his methods and records will not be clear and easy to determine. Remember, what seems overwhelming in the first six months to a year becomes second nature from thereon. Be patient and don't be hard on yourself.

You will have to sort through your financial affairs and organize them according to your individual needs. That means finding your own "envelopes" or ledger sheets. Get a handle on your financial position now so that you know where you stand today and in the future. If this requires that you find someone to help you get organized and manage, then do just that.

Any correctable positions of your financial situation should be corrected sooner rather than later.

Money will not "work" by itself.

You need to make the decisions necessary to make your money work for you — and the sooner the better. Those decisions can be best facilitated — and made more wisely — with the help of a qualified financial advisor.

Summary — Chapter 8

1. Understand the position in which you were left.
2. Sort out your financial affairs and organize them according to your individual needs.
3. Make necessary corrections to your financial situation sooner rather then later.
4. Seek or employ a qualified financial advisor to help you make your money work for you.

HELPFUL WEBSITES:

www.leapsystems.com

Staying abreast with a constantly changing world is a difficult task. Of the numerous money decisions that you will face and must make, choosing which ones are right for you can be complex and very time consuming. Also, information overload can lead to indecision and fincial paralysis.

The LEAP SYSTEM® empowers you to take full control and overcome the complexity of the financial world by providing easy to understand, easy to follow, and easy to implement financial models and strategies.

CHAPTER 9

Your New Life: Prioritizing, Banking, Budgeting and Planning for Your Future.

"It was comforting to know that I could pick up the phone and call one of my sons," my mother would say.

Establishing Priorities

Mary L. came to me a year after her husband died. Although she had been making financial decisions — some better than others — for most of that year, her approach had been haphazard and she found herself experiencing more and more dissatisfaction with her situation.

"I thought this was supposed to get easier," she said in a warm, engaging voice. She had a quick smile and a determination to improve herself and her family. "I mean, after the first couple of months.. the kids were great. Very supportive. I have two girls, one in college, the other with a young family of her own."

"I went back to school. Took some interesting classes. I've enjoyed learning a little bit about computers. I'm only fifty-two. I still have some productive years left..."

"I just have the sense that things are getting away from me." She settled back in the chair, looking both tired and bewildered.

"Sometimes one of the hardest things any of us has to do is to prioritize our own lives," I told her. (Many times, people make decisions to be in charge of a situation. Unfortunately, if their decisions are arbitrary, even taking charge becomes defeating.)

"Let me ask you a question. What is important to you?"

Mary crossed her arms across her chest and thought for a moment. "My health. My girls." She looked at me. "The house. I enjoy my house and my garden."

"I assume you still support your daughter in college. Do you still give financial assistance to your married daughter?"

"We, my husband and I, helped them secure their mortgage. I will still contribute two hundred dollars a month to help them with their payments. I also have to help with the day-care costs."

As we spoke, a clearer picture of Mary's needs and wants began to emerge. The one thing I tried to impress her with was the understanding that the number one priority had to be herself, then came all other family obligations.

I helped her list her financial obligations using List 2, 3 and 4. Then we spoke about plans to achieve the desired financial goals she had for herself. (This is the cornerstone of the financial plan which I will cover in the next section.)

As we spoke, I learned that Mary had always wanted to tour the art museums in Europe.

"Perhaps a dream," she sighed.

"Not necessarily," I pointed out. There was nothing unreasonable or extravagant about arranging Mary's finances in such a way that she would be able to enjoy such a trip.

"Oh, I don't know," she said when I explained how she could do it. "I've always been such a practical person. That's why I'm taking computer classes."

"There is nothing wrong with being practical," I told her. "In fact, I admire it. You should also treat yourself to the things you enjoy. Perhaps a dinner out, theater, or why not art classes. Or maybe a trip to Europe."

That summer, I received a postcard from Florence, Italy. Mary wrote that she was having a wonderful time.

"Thank you," she added. "It's not that I couldn't have done it without you, it's just that the likelihood is, I wouldn't have. I don't know if I ever would have figured it out without help."

Before you sit down with your financial advisor you should take time to think about a set of objectives and goals for yourself. What do you want to accomplish with your financial situation? What would you like to do if you were able to do anything you wanted? Think about your "wish list" and your "pragmatic list."

Once you have a clear sense of what your goals are, then you should sit down with the most qualified advisor to devise the appropriate strategy\plan that would allow you to realize these goals. While insurance professionals and accountants are fine advisors and certainly well-qualified to devise a financial plan, a financial planner (macro manager) is generally your best choice because he or she is best positioned to oversee all aspects of your financial well-being.

For starters, make sure that any financial planner with whom you consider working is a Chartered Financial Consultant (ChFC), Certified Financial Planner (CFP), or an accountant — preferably a CPA with a Personal Financial Specialist (PFS) designation. These certifications represent your best guarantee that the person you go to for advice is competent to give you sound and safe financial guidance.

Your financial planner should be your central advisor, the captain of your financial team. Your planner will prepare an overview of your entire situation and help guide you through all aspects of your financial life. He or she will be able to take into account your "wish list," modifying where necessary, making it real for you where possible.

Your first goal should be to maintain a standard of living that will enable you to enjoy a comfortable life style. That should include travel, movies, dining, and other pleasures you enjoy. In addition, you should have a financial plan that will afford you security in the event of emergencies such as illness. Many people even prepay their funeral and cemetery expenses. I'll discuss this in more detail later.

You should also consider charitable contributions that you would like to continue or begin. In addition, your financial plan should account for any professional assistance you might seek — financial or personal.

Remember, everyone's objectives are different. One of my clients insisted that her financial arrangements must allow her to continue living in her house. Others were better served by selling their homes and moving into apartments or condominiums.

Important preferences should be factored into your plan. Remember, in order to achieve a financial plan that satisfies you, you will have to be honest about your needs.

"To thine own self be true" is another well-worn phrase deserving of repetition here. Know what you want and need. That will make it much easier for a financial planner to help you.

Remember, your financial plan is NOT carved in stone. It is, at best, a map to guide you along your financial journey. Just like any other journey, detours, changes in the terrain, and things that catch our interest, cause us to adjust our route. Your advisor should be there to help you negotiate these changes.

When You Are Ready, To Whom Should You Turn?

In spite of news reports touting statistics that suggest that the family as we know it is becoming obsolete, the fact of the matter is that we all rely on a network of relatives and friends for support. While the "traditional" nuclear family has borne the brunt of economic, social, and geographic changes in our country, it is still going strong. More to the point, the "new family" of step-siblings, half-siblings, in-laws, etc., also provides for deep, enriching and loving relationships.

In times of trouble and stress, we should all still be able to turn to our families. That should certainly be the case when it is time for you to begin to explore your financial options.

You should consider consulting first with family members who have some business experience. No, this does not mean that you must have an uncle or brother-in-law who is a Chief Executive Officer of a major Wall Street firm. What it means is that you need someone you can trust to have your best interests at heart to begin the process of sorting out the various options you have available to you. Some experience and knowledge of investments would be a great benefit.

Anne's son-in-law was the middle-level manager of a stationery supply corporation. Although most people would not have thought of him as the first person for her to discuss financial matters with after her husband died, she found him to be the most helpful — and accessible.

"He just has a good head on his shoulders," Anne said. "I knew he wouldn't tell me to do something that was foolish. I trusted him. He helped me get my feet on solid ground."

When Anne explained to me what exactly her son-in-law had done, I felt the desire to applaud his good sense. Basically, he walked her through the difficult emotional period and listened to her and understood her financial goals; in essence, how much she needed each month to live. Then, when she was a bit more prepared to face decisions, he helped her work through her paperwork.

When her needs reached a point where she needed someone with more expertise, he told her so. He also promised to be with her when she interviewed professionals to work with.

"It's not that he told me so much," Anne said. "But what he did tell me was sensible and he got me started."

Anne had the benefit of a trusted member of the family to help her. Hopefully, your family has some good advisors who are familiar with your husband's financial situation. If, however, there is no one in your family with whom you feel comfortable turning to, or if you do not have family with you, then you should find an advisor who you are comfortable with and who you can trust. Trust is the key issue! I will mention this again and again. You must trust your advisor.

You will, of course, want to consult with someone who is very knowledgeable and competent to deal with your financial situation.

First Advisors

In addition to your family, your "first advisors" should be your accountant, who handled your previous tax return, and your lawyer, who handled your husband's Will. These two should work together to guarantee that all assets in your husband's estate are accounted for. In most cases, this is a very straightforward process. The assets that your attorney is unaware of are generally known to your accountant. Together, they can "fit all the pieces" together.

If need be, a financial planner, like myself, who not only sees the big picture, but is familiar with reading an income tax return, can be of some assistance in "working backwards" to discover missing assets. Remember, sometimes your husband's advisors were privy to all of his business dealings.

Again, you should consult with a professional you feel most comfortable with. As I'll mention later in the "Closing the Estate" chapter, I strongly recommend that you consult with an attorney who specializes in tax law (trusts and estates).

You should no more expect a general practice or criminal law attorney to be able to advise you in this process than you would expect a pediatrician to perform brain surgery. There are times when specialization should be respected.

This is one of those times.

Trust and expertise are vital in selecting your attorney. Estate tax law is a highly specialized field which must be taken care of properly to avoid problems. Do not let an attorney or any other advisor unfamiliar with the surrogate procedure take on this responsibility. You have too much to lose and too much time that can be wasted. This is very important and should not be taken lightly.

Louise told me about her uncle's estate. "It was not a tremendous estate," she said. "A nice home. A few modest investments. He was a nice man, my uncle. Successful but not spectacularly so."

"Anyway, my uncle had a friend, an attorney who specialized in criminal law. My aunt turned to him after my uncle died."

"Do you know that my uncle's estate took a year to probate?" She shook her head in amazement. "The way the process dragged on made my aunt very upset."

A drawn-out probate process is always aggravating for the family. It is always more costly. And it is almost always unnecessary.

Second Opinion

While it might appear excessive when negotiating financial strategies, second opinions can be vital. My strong recommendation is that you have more than one advisor, and in the absence of a second advisor, at least get a second opinion — regardless of how "simple and straightforward" your situation is.

If you have more than one child, you'll be able to get that second opinion without too much difficulty. The difficulty might be in getting your children to agree on a single financial strategy.

My mother was fortunate to have two caring and loving sons when my father died. Though my brother and I were not always able to ease our mother's concerns, we were always there for each other. Together we made decisions to choose our advisors.

A good advisor is one who listens. A good advisor can also be a family member or a good friend that you have confidence in.

While financial advice is absolutely necessary from the person to whom you seek guidance, emotional support is another important facet of the relationship. One of my favorite clients, a woman who was widowed several years ago, always used to greet me with the same question, "Why am I so afraid?"

I always tried to reassure her that her financial situation was really very sound and that she had nothing to worry about, but my words seemed to have little effect on her feelings. This troubled me for a long time until I began to see the same fear — implicitly and explicitly — from many other widows.

I learned from these women that, in addition to the sound advice I give them, one of the greatest services I can provide is to assure them that they are secure both *financially* and *emotionally.*

These women are not going to spend all their money; thanks to a wise and experienced financial advisor.

A good financial advisor understands that planning is not solely a question of adding and subtracting dollars and cents. A financial advisor needs to understand you and your fears as well as your needs and dreams. A majority of my time is often spent on the client's personal problems, including children and grandchildren, and if the widow is young enough, her parents. The expression "sandwich generation" is sometimes mentioned to describe when there are both parents and children to worry about.

These family problems are important for your advisor and you to understand each other. It is important for you to connect with your advisor and feel a close relationship.

How we manage and spend our money is very telling about the kind of people we are. No financial advisor should see you as little more than a balance sheet. You are more than the sum of your assets. You deserve to have that understood and respected.

One of my clients still frets and fears about running out of money, food and household items. Her freezer is overstocked with too much food. Her household supplies are four deep in her cabinets.

I gently kid her about these things. It doesn't hurt to find a financial advisor who has a sense of humor — and who understands how to use that humor to continually strengthen the relationship that you have.

The Team Approach

It is most important to be able to make sure that the different advisors communicate effectively with one another. They should each understand their role and responsibility, as well as the roles and responsibilities of others you have come to rely upon.

The advisors that commonly work together are:

Accountant
Lawyer

Investment Advisor - primarily specializes in investments

Financial Planner\Insurance Agent - does the financial plan and can also sell insurance (life and health) and investments

Of course there is some overlap but each of these roles is appropriately handled by a separate individual.

A good financial planner will help coordinate all your other advisors. You will find that, at first, you will need some of these professionals more than the others, particularly the lawyer. But, as time goes on, your financial planner, accountant, and investment advisor will be the people you call with a specific question or concern as it arises. If your financial planner is good, he or she will tell you who else you need to call when your question is out of his or her domain.

One client of mine always dreamed of taking an Alaskan cruise but she felt silly sharing that dream with an earlier advisor. "I thought he would wonder why someone like me wanted to go to Alaska?" Consequently, although her financial portfolio remained healthy, she was let to believe she could not take this trip. She certainly could have! I suggested certain changes in her investments which would allow her to travel without compromising her security.

Her investments had done better than we projected. She planned another trip, this time to the Far East.

"I always wanted to walk along the Great Wall of China," she told me with a faraway, dreamy quality in her voice.

There is no need to worry about how to find an advisor you can trust. Simply trust your feelings. You'll be able to tell right away if you can establish a successful and honest relationship with an advisor. You'll know by the way the advisor speaks to you and how you are treated.

On issues of trust, go with your "gut".

Fees

Don't shy away from an advisor because of fees or commissions. The advisor is a true professional and should earn a fee or commission as compensation for the value and service that he or she provide for you. It is not unusual for an advisor to earn both a fee and a commission as long as it is predetermined and disclosed.

Don't get blind-sided by financial planners who call themselves "fee only" planners. Good planners who collect fees as well as commissions, by law, must present a generic plan without mentioning a specific product. You have the option of buying products from that planner after the plan is presented. Most people end up buying from that planner since the planner knows the individual's situation very well and would rather deal with one person. Others deal with the planner strictly on a fee basis. Either one is acceptable. Be wary of planners and investment advisors who have a limited supply of products and urge you to buy one specific product.

"Penny wise, pound foolish."

"You get what you pay for."

There are hundreds of truisms when it comes to how you manage your money. In the case of advisors, they are especially true.

A trusted advisor is worth many times what he or she gets paid.

You want to feel — and be — reassured that your financial health is sound. The professional cost for such reassurance is always well worth it.

Financial health and peace of mind frees you to accomplish so much more in your life. Knowing that your finances are taken care of empowers you to focus on other areas of your life, areas that could provide you with tremendous enjoyment.

You WANT to be independent. Not only financially independent but independent of the worry and stress of ensuring your financial independence. One of the primary goals in settling on a financial advisor is finding one who will make you feel comfortable in "letting go" of that worry and stress.

For this reason, you should ask friends for the names and numbers of their financial advisors. Speak with them. Get an objective assessment of how successful their financial relationship is.

As an example, most of my clients who are widows have been referred to me by their children. I take this as the ultimate compliment that I am accomplishing everything I need to accomplish as a financial advisor.

Although you might be anxious to "get everything settled," and to allow your advisor to assume the burden of your finances, I would advise you to take those first steps a bit more slowly and cautiously. "Haste makes waste" is another expression that is appropriate to our discussion. You do not have to suffer through bad experiences with advisors before finding the right one.

Be selective. Find a qualified financial advisor who you can trust.

How Often Should You Meet With Your Advisors?

You should meet with your financial advisor whenever your personal situation changes. A new grandchild. A child purchasing a house. If your situation changes, you should find out whether there are any financial, tax, or legal arrangements which need to be adjusted.

Some professionals, such as lawyers, accountants, or financial planners, can be retained for periodic meetings to review your situation with you. If your advisor offers such an arrangement, consider taking advantage of it. Find your "contact" comfort level and keep on top of your financial well-being.

Before we move on to some particulars on planning for your future, remember the following key items:

1. Your number one priority has to be yourself!
2. Set desirable financial goals.
3. With the help of a qualified financial planner, devise an appropriate strategy\plan to realize your goals.
4. Work with a team of financial advisers who you can trust.

HELPFUL WEBSITES For choosing a financial advisor;

www.theamericancollege.edu/consumer-resources/find-an-advisor

www.fpanet.org/plannersearch/search.cfm

www.sec.gov/investor/brokers.htm

Banking and Budgeting - A Key to Accomplishing Financial Well-Being

Savings

You want to have savings. How much savings should you have? Fifty percent of your income should be in conservative savings vehicles such as savings accounts, certificate of deposits, money market accounts, fixed annuities and cash value life insurance.

Not only are these funds readily available, but they become your foundation. Once you have at least fifty percent in savings, then you can start moving future savings into "rules based" plans such as IRAs or retirement plans. The next savings dollars should be directed into bonds (government, corporate and municipals), then equities (preferred stock, blue chip stocks and growth securities) and then real estate (rental property) and finally, collectibles or a business.

Paying Bills

Paying bills is a demanding reality of managing your own financial affairs. My best advice regarding bill paying is to minimize the number of days you have to devote to this task.

As much as possible, pay your bills once or twice a month — preferably on the first and fifteen of that month. Several bills may have to be attended to on other days, the fewer days you spend on paying bills, the more free time you will have for yourself. If your money is making money, send it at the last possible day.

Mortgage bills, credit card bills, telephone, utility and insurance bills should be paid when they are received.

You do not want to invite additional charges in the form of late fees. You also do not want to damage your credit rating.

As I've previously noted, it is a good idea to review your situation a few months later. At that time, you will be able to more objectively assess how you are faring. You might want to consider doing this with your accountant, financial planner, or family advisor. At that time, you can discuss how you have been paying your bills, what changes you'd like to make, and how best to devise a method that is most satisfying to you, while still meeting all your financial needs and obligations. One possibility is to have the payment automatically deducted from your check book. Another is hiring a bill-paying service or online banking.

While you should document and file the payment of some bills (see Chapter 6 on "Getting Organized" for setting up a filing and record keeping system) — mortgage, car payments, medical, etc. — there are other bills which do not demand such attention or filing. Magazine subscriptions are a good example of this second kind of bill. (See next box about subscriptions.) Make sure to jot down the invoice number on your check along with the time period which your payment covers. Now you can throw out the invoice, eliminate duplicate paperwork, and have the canceled check as proof of your payment.

Magazines keep billing and start early, so keep magazine subscriptions on file by canceled check because they ask for payment 6 months prior to the end. You can clip the address label that has the expiration of the subscription date and attach it to the check.

Car insurance. Health insurance. Long-term care insurance. These will all need to be evaluated and adjusted. Meet with your insurance agent as soon as you are comfortable to review your insurance portfolio to assess your current needs. Remember there are often different insurance professionals for each type of insurance. Follow the same rules with insurance advisors as I previously mentioned in this chapter when selecting advisors.

For example, with your life insurance, make sure you seek expert advice from an individual agent who is licensed and who specializes in helping you organize this very important area. Don't necessarily use your auto or homeowner's agent for the other insurance I've mentioned. Be sure to review who the beneficiaries are of your life insurance plan.

I will speak more completely on the issue of beneficiaries and owners of life insurance policies later in this section on "Estate Planning."

Don't let the "I" word intimidate you — especially when it comes to life insurance and long term care insurance. Both have a place and could be of significant benefit, if you qualify, in protecting and providing for your family. (I will also explain insurance further in Part II.)

HELPFUL WEBSITES:

For paying bills;

www.clearcheckbook.com

Check and Budget Your Expenses

"How will I know what my expenses are going to be?"

If your husband paid all the bills, the chances are you do not have a clear idea of your cost of living. You therefore may not be able to know all your expenses. Every month, you will receive your canceled checks from your bank.

Go through those checks. In this way, you will learn all the necessary living expenses. You will also know your fixed costs, monthly payments, and all other obligations. This will help you budget, or estimate your ongoing expenditures.

You might want to examine canceled checks over the course of several months in order to "average" these varying expenses. You will see that over time you'll be able to estimate quite closely your monthly grocery costs, utility costs, out-of-pocket expenses, etc.

In the beginning, you might want to go through this process fairly regularly — weekly or monthly. However, as you and your finances settle into a comfortable relationship, you will find that updating these lists is only necessary on a yearly basis.

It is often necessary to sit down with your accountant, financial planner, or family advisor when you review and revise this list. Over time, you can use my lists 2, 3 & 4 to see how your expenses are doing. If you find your expenses are rising, try to determine why.

Interestingly, not all "expenses" are bad. In fact, some actually reduce your liabilities.

With certain expenses, such as a mortgage, part of the monthly payment is a repayment of your mortgage balance. Because of this, over time, the mortgage balance is reduced and eliminated. The other part of the mortgage payment — interest — will become progressively smaller as the mortgage is paid off. Because of these kinds of "expenses," some women are actually debt free when their husbands pass away.

Periodic reviews of your mortgage interest rate is important to determine if the interest rate you are being charged is comparable to interest rates being offered on new mortgages. Check with a banker or a mortgage broker regarding what new rates are available. With the help of one of your advisors, such as your accountant or financial planner, you can determine if the closing costs associated with "refinancing" your mortgage should be incurred to get a lower interest rate. Closing costs can also be borrowed and added to your mortgage balance.

Some women benefit from mortgage life insurance which their husbands may have taken out. If so, then the mortgage holder should be aware of the situation and the mortgage is "satisfied" and eliminated immediately.

The best case scenario is, of course, to be left "debt free" and "mortgage free." Unfortunately, for many women that is not the case. Becoming a widow too often poses a real threat to continuing the lifestyle you have enjoyed. This is why it might be recommended that you use life insurance proceeds to pay off any debt, including your mortgage. This is a good idea particularly if you are paying a higher interest expense than your money can earn as an investment. Some old and current first mortgages are at reasonably low interest rates and should be kept. In addition, these interest costs maybe currently income tax deductible. (Check with your accountant if all your mortgage interest is tax deductible.) Credit card debt and personal loans or bank lines of credit should be paid off as soon as possible because they tend to have extremely high interest rates and are not tax deductible. (Unless they are for business purposes.)

If you are were left with too little money to live, and own

your own home, you can consider a reverse mortgage. A reverse mortgage is basically selling your house to the bank. (They get the house after you die.) The bank turns around and gives you an income stream and the right to live in the house for life. When I reviewed this option for a client, it was better to sell the house and live off the proceeds. Check with your financial advisor to see which option works best for you.

With patience, understanding and guidance, it is possible to have your financial situation improve during this next phase of your life. I will discuss this a bit later in Part II, on "Planning For The Future."

Summary — Chapter 9

1. You want to have savings.
2. Keep time required for paying bills to a minimum.
3. Check your expenses to determine what your cash flow needs are, including income tax payments.

HELPFUL WEBSITES:

For budgeting;

http://financialplan.about.com/msubbudg.htm

For reverse mortgages;

www.reversemortgage.org

For refinancing an existing mortgage;

www.mortgageloan.com

CHAPTER 10

Your Husband's Will

"The lawyers did a good job in explaining to us what all our options were," my mother pointed out to us.

"I don't know why, but I was apprehensive to have my husband's Will read," Lee, another of my clients, confessed to me. "Maybe it was all those TV movies..."

Television doesn't always portray real life accurately. That was certainly true in this case — and in most cases of the administration and processing of a Will. Lee had an image of the family gathering in a solemn ceremony in a judge or attorney's office. The Will would be opened and then read, providing startling revelations into her husband's life. Clearly, that did not happen. More to the point, it is a myth. Not only is there no such thing as "reading the Will," but there is no legal requirement that the Will has to be read.

In fact, your husband's Will might not have as much importance as you think. This is good to remember in case you have difficulty locating it.

The importance of the Will is directly related to your list of assets, liabilities and life insurance policies. For example, if you were a joint owner with your husband with rights of survivorship, you would automatically inherit the property or properties that you own already. So too if you are a direct beneficiary of an IRA, pension, 401(k) plan, or life insurance policy.

All of these assets are non-probatable. This means they pass outside of the Will.

Only those assets in your husband's name alone are subject to his Will. The only other way in which assets may pass through his Will is if an asset had the beneficiary designation of his estate, such as a life insurance policy. This would have been done for estate planning purposes. I will discuss this later as well.

I am getting ahead of myself, however. While the Will itself, might not be as important a legal document as you may have thought, it still bears the potential for problems, delays and costs. Make sure your attorney is a specialist. In addition, you want this specialist to be available to explain certain terms or eventualities, such as creation of trusts.

Trusts Under Your Husband's Will

Two of the most popular trusts created today are the unified credit shelter trust or the "bypass trust" and the "Q-tip" trust.

The "bypass trust" was set up primarily as an estate tax reduction technique. Hopefully, you were left as a co-trustee with a child or family friend, primarily so you have some say in where the monies will be invested and who will ultimately inherit these assets. Generally, there are certain rules that need to be followed to access the principal. Usually, you are entitled to all the income the trust earns.

The same basic rules of life insurance trusts apply to these trusts — regarding checking accounts, income, and keeping the trusts out of your estate and taxed upon your own death. (See Chapter 4 under Life Insurance for more about life insurance trusts.)

One of my clients, Fran, kept on asking about taking principal from the "bypass" trust. "Should I take the amount over and above the original amount that was in the trust?" she said a few years after her husband's passing. I advised her that she could, if she wanted to, under the rules of the trust. She was better off, however, depleting her own assets first, since the assets in her own name, if large enough, would be taxed at her subsequent death where the trust would not. She finally understood that what her husband had set up, was the smart thing at that time. Remember, not only the original principal, but also the appreciation of the principal, no matter how large it gets, avoids estate taxes. If you have a choice of what asset goes in the trust after your husband's death, it should be the asset with the most growth potential.

The other trust, the "Q-tip" trust, is primarily set up to provide all income to you and give you access to principal when needed. This trust is not merely for estate planning purposes, but also to guarantee that upon your remarriage and ultimate death, your children will inherit the money.

The humorous reason I heard that this trust was created by Congress, was to make sure that the politicians who had multiple marriages would ensure that their children of previous marriages would inherit their money and not their former wife's new husband.

The other reason I've heard, was to enable the deceased husband to "rule from the grave" and keep the money intact, preventing the money from being squandered. Money in your own name can be spent freely and has no restrictions. Money in the name of the trust has some limitations which you'll need to learn in order to possibly adjust to having someone else as a trustee. This is where good legal advice is key.

Rearranging Accounts — What you Can and Cannot Correct!

The only accounts you will have immediate access to are those that were either joint accounts or accounts in your name only. Any account in your husband's name alone will have to go through the courts before it can be changed to your name. Certain checks made payable to your husband may also have to go through his estate account.

Some accounts, such as retirement plans and IRAs, are more accessible since only a death certificate is required before the account can be changed into your name alone. However, even in these "more accessible" accounts, be prepared for frustrations. Financial institutions are very "picky" when it comes to forms and filling them out perfectly. Until the legal requirements are met, some accounts simply cannot be adjusted.

Revocable Living Trusts

If your husband set up a revocable living trust and there were assets transferred into the trust, you will have immediate access if you were named as the beneficiary or successor trustee. This can make for a very smooth transition or no transition at all depending on what assets are in the name of the living trust. (That was the main reason for it to be done.) After your husband dies, the trust becomes irrevocable and cannot be changed.

If you do not have your own revocable living trust and you have assets in your own name, you might want to consider such a trust. I'll discuss this, and other options later in Part II on "Planning For The Future."

Summary — Chapter 10

1. Certain joint property and beneficiary designation property does not go through the Will.
2. The "bypass" trust was a smart move by your husband, since it potentially will save your family estate taxes.
3. A "Q-tip" trust will avoid the need for a pre-nuptial agreement if you remarry.
4. To avoid delays, make sure all papers are filled out correctly when assets are being transferred to your name.
5. A "revocable" trust avoids probate and makes the transition to carrying on with your financial life seamless.

CHAPTER 11

Closing The Estate

"It was such a relief when the final estate tax return was filed and all the estate accounts were closed," my mother stated.

Even though this is a difficult emotional time, it is an important time to begin trusting your instincts. If you are uncomfortable with someone for any reason, do not work with them when it comes to choosing an attorney for closing the estate. The decisions you will be making could have a tremendous impact on your future and the future of your family. You owe it to yourself to seek the most competent advice you can while working with people you trust and like. Let me repeat that. You owe it to yourself to seek the most competent advice you can while working with people you trust and like.

One of the hardest things one has to do is to be assertive in terms of our personal preferences — especially when dealing with professional people.

Most attorneys who are generalists do not recommend an attorney who is a specialist in Wills and estates. General practitioner attorneys think this is an opportunity to gouge for fees. Make sure you get a written agreement and understanding of what the legal fees and court costs are first — before you hire an attorney.

Always remember, you are in charge. It is your life. If you hire a lawyer — or any other professional — you have the right to fire that lawyer.

If you anticipate difficulties — or if you are already experiencing difficulties — get legal and financial advice on your own and always, always keep solid documentation to back up your problems.

"I am pleased to say I was able to make decisions based on my husband's Will," Lee told me. "I had a friend who wasn't in charge and it was terrible."

Hopefully you, like Lee, were left in charge as executrix of your husband's Will. If you were not named to execute the Will then hopefully one of your children was. If you and your children are asked to serve as executrix or executor (masculine form of executrix) then, by law, executor fees are set. In a family situation, executor fees are generally waived. However, there may be a tax benefit to receive executor fees. Check with your attorney to see if there is an advantage for executor fees to be paid. If a non-family member was left in charge, they have the option of waiving the executor fee or receiving it.

If you were not left as an executrix or trustee, you may be in for a surprise.

One of my clients, Zelda, was not named as executrix or as trustee which resulted in a loss of control, particularly because two attorneys were made executors and trustees. Since all the money was left in trust, the trustees had to be consulted on everything before Zelda had access to the money. This was an ironic position for her husband to have left her in because she was an expert in the stock market with years of experience in investing. Her hands were tied however and she could not control her own destiny. Once a person dies, the Will becomes law.

Remember this when it comes to drafting your own Will.

The executrix or executor is responsible for the estate. He or she is legally empowered to make fundamental decisions about the estate. Depending on their knowledge — or the ability of the advisors they select — the process could be short and simple or long and agonizing. One responsibility of the executrix is investing the money in the estate during the administration period. This is generally a short time period, so treasuries or money markets would be appropriate.

The executor or executrix of a Will has some other specific obligations which must be met, besides to follow the wishes of the Will. Among these are: paying debts, taxes and expenses, in addition to identifying all assets at their current value. (Remember to check with the Veterans Administration if your husband was a veteran, to see if any benefits were due him.)

As executrix, you should know that a probate process may need to be done. This all depends on what the assets arc. In Latin, "probate" means "to prove." Certain items must be proved to the court before assets can be distributed or specific bequests made. The court that takes care of this process is called the Surrogate Court. Your tax attorney will direct you through this process. Your tax attorney will also direct you if any federal or state estate tax returns need to be filed and what, if any, taxes must be paid. I'll discuss some of these issues later in Part II "Planning For The Future."

Initially, what you want to know and understand is that, depending on the Will and the assets owned, an estate has been started and the final accounting must be done. This accounting is not only for assets but for income as well. The key date is day of death. For example, earned income that is received prior to death is on a decedent's income tax return. This is a key distinction which will help you understand that the advisor is just following the rules and not making them up to do extra work.

Income from a regular salary, for example, will not require a separate accounting. Your husband's employer will notify you with your husband's total earnings for the year and will stop paying him at his death, unless he had an employment contract. If your husband received income from some other source or if he was self-employed, this situation becomes more complicated. I have previously discussed this under "What did your husband do for a living" in Chapter 4 on "Uncovering Your Husband's Financial Records." Needless to say, if you encounter this, you should consult with a qualified accountant or tax attorney. He or she will also instruct you on how to account for the expenses of your husband's estate, offsetting any income subject to either income or estate taxes.

Done properly, the probate process can move simply and quickly. Your goal is to facilitate such an efficient conclusion to the process.

Common causes of delay in the probate process are: the inability to find the original Will, inability to find distributees or witnesses, and the incapacity of a distributee and a child contesting a Will. (The last one is the least common of them all.) Probate can be avoided with a living trust. See Chapter 17 on "Estate Planning" to learn more about the use of living trusts.

Summary — Chapter 11

1. Seek competent and trustworthy people to help you close the estate.
2. Use a specialist.
3. If you are the executrix, remember you are in charge.

"Denial is over, shock is diminished, and realization of "this is it" sets in and depression must be fought," is the experience my mother expressed.

CHAPTER 12

What if You Become Ill?

"The best laid plans..." is the literary version of Murphy's Law.

Should you become ill, your entire investment strategy can be rendered ineffectual. In order to avoid this, you should protect yourself with the right insurance package.

Health insurance is a must. If you are sixty-five years of age, you are eligible for Medicare. Medicare is administered by the federal government and can be reached at the same number for social security information at 1-800-772-1213. If you are under sixty-five, you must provide your own policy or continue under your husband's policy if possible.

If you are sixty-five and are on Medicare, you should consider a Medicare supplement policy called a "Medigap" policy. Medigap policies are available through private insurance companies and cover almost everything Medicare does not, with the notable exception of long-term care for nursing homes and home health care.

Consequently, you should consider a long-term care policy. Such a policy can help defray the costs associated with home care if you find yourself unable to perform some of your daily activities. In addition, if you find yourself having to go into a senior's residence — either a nursing home or an assisted living facility — your policy will reduce your out-of-pocket costs.

Each policy offers different options and features. Examine the features you are comfortable with and weigh them against what you are able to afford. Premiums can run between $1,000 and $10,000 depending on what age you take out the policy. The earlier you take out the policy the better. One of my old friends told me about his dad, who keep putting off buying the insurance. By the time he needed it, it was too late. He was sick.

A client of mine recently lost her husband after he was in a nursing home for four years. It cost her over $8,000 a month! (That's close to $400,000.) When I told her there was insurance that would have covered that cost, she told me, "I would stand up in a room full of people and tell them to get that insurance!" I should take her up on that in my next seminar. It was very convincing.

If you do not have long-term care insurance because you can not qualify medically or financially for it, your only option would be to apply for Medicaid. If you qualify, medically and financially, then your state government will cover the costs of your stay.

Some states offer partnership plans with Medicaid so you don't have to divest yourself of all your assets to qualify for Medicaid.

If you can afford it, long term care insurance should be seriously considered. It can help you avoid dependency on others and retain your freedom of choice. In addition, the premiums may be deducted on your income tax return as medical expenses. Check with your financial advisor to see if you qualify and what the best policy is for you. Only go with a reputable company that is highly rated by independent rating agencies such as A.M. Best.

Summary — Chapter 12

1. You can be wiped out financially without the right health or long term care insurance.
2. Seek an insurance specialist for health or long term care insurance.

HELPFUL WEBSITES:

Social Security–Medicare;

www.ssa.gov

Shoppers guide to long term care insurance;

www.ltcfeds.com/documents/files/NAIC_Shoppers_Guide.PDF

CHAPTER 13

Planning For The Inevitable

Making Final Arrangements

Ultimately, all our considerations have danced around a most sensitive topic — either the loss of your husband or your own eventual death. Few things address this reality as directly as prepaid funeral and final resting place arrangements.

Let the funeral home know what your wishes are. If your final arrangements deal with burial arrangements, here are a few important items you should check on;

- The deed or proof of ownership document. If you don't have documentation, verify records with the cemetery.
- If your spouse was buried within the grounds of Burial Society, Family Circle or religious organization; be sure to protect your "right of interment" to a specific gravesite. Get it in writing and keep the document.
- Make sure the person who will be arranging your affairs has a copy of the documentation.

Some additional items for consideration if not already addressed are;

- Since cemeteries have different rules and regulations regulating the size and type of memorial stone permitted to mark gravesites; ask the cemetery or monument dealer for assistance.
- Since cemeteries are forever, it is suggested to make arrangements for perpetual or endowed care. Such arrangements can be provided as a codicil in a will. Get details from the cemetery and provide them to your attorney.

As difficult as this subject is to address — there are such obvious benefits to making such arrangements, both financial and emotional, that it is worth the discomfort of confronting the subject head-on.

Certain funeral homes will guarantee the cost if a pre-paid funeral is arranged. The only additional costs your family will deal with are outside costs such as religious services, and cemetery charges (opening up a grave).

Of course, by making your own arrangements, you are also saving your surviving family members the emotional upheaval of having to make decisions at that very difficult time.

Your investment in final arrangements is relatively risk-free. While you are alive, you can revoke your arrangements at your discretion, including a move to another state. However, your family can revoke what you've set up after you die. In other words, your family is not bound to follow your wishes. You can also express your wishes in a separate letter that you keep with your original will, which can include final arrangements. (This also is not legally binding, so you have to hope that your children will honor your last request).

Monies left with the funeral home will earn interest that you may be required to accumulate in your account which can be used by the funeral home to offset any inflationary increases. This interest is income taxable even though you are not receiving the interest.

Monies left with cemeteries for perpetual care by law are protected and are regulated by the state; only the interest can be used and not the principal. Make sure the person arranging your final affairs is aware of what has been done.

The cemetery has the right to ask for additional funds if the investment income from the perpetual care endowment is not enough for that year to cover the cost of maintenance. The good news is that by state law the cemetery has to still maintain the grave and that no additional funds need to be paid.

Not-for-profit cemeteries in the state of New York, for example, are regulated by the New York State Cemetery Board (NY Dept. of State) and must file an annual financial report with the state. Cemeteries are subject to both inspection and audit. A prospective consumer of cemetery services can ask the cemetery to see its financials. With respect to perpetual care endowments, families can ask for an annual accounting of income and expenses in order to determine the adequacy of the endowment for their account (whether it be a single gravesite or a family plot).

As always, ask questions and get the answers in writing.

Prepaid funeral arrangements are also regulated by state law where the funeral home is located. If your funeral ends up costing less than the money that was prepaid, the funeral home must, under certain state laws, refund the difference to your family. Check with the funeral director to see what the state law is before you prepay. Certain states will not refund the money if the funeral costs less than the actual money you prepay.

Summary — Chapter 13

1. Prepaid funeral and final resting place arrangements will make it much easier on your family during a very difficult time.

HELPFUL WEBSITES:

NY State Association of Cemeteries;

www.nysac.com

NY State Funeral Directors Association;

www.nysfda.org

CHAPTER 14

Investment Planning

"I really trusted my investment advisor," my mother said in a reassuring tone.

Who Should Set Up Your Investment Plan?

You might already have existing investments. You may have advisors who have been involved in your investment strategy. If this is the case, you should sit down with them as soon as possible for a thorough review of your investment portfolio. It is very likely that your current portfolio will have to be adjusted to meet your new life requirements.

When your husband was working, income from his and your investments was "icing on the cake." His earnings allowed you to maintain your lifestyle. Now, however, these investments will have to provide you with more of the substance of your day-to-day financial needs.

Even if you are working, the investments will have to work harder for you, if your financial circumstances are to remain healthy.

Betty continued to work after her husband died. "Bob was what I would call semi-retired. He had been an accountant himself and so was able to continue some accounts. He worked during tax season but not like he had done during his younger years."

"Still, after he was gone I realized, although small, just how important this income was. The difference between one and two incomes is so dramatic. Today, not too many people can manage on a single income."

Betty was fortunate. As an accountant, her husband had

made prudent, conservative investments over the years. These investments came to represent a significant value. Her portfolio needed to be adjusted, however, so that part of these investments would earn income she needed for daily living.

With some considerate decisions, some of the money was reallocated into areas that were still quite safe, but which earned higher interest. In a short time, her investments were working for her, offsetting the loss of Bob's income.

Even with a more successful investment package, I counseled Betty not to be too hasty to stop working. In addition to being a source of income, work gave her a very important social outlet. If nothing else, it gave her some place to go and get her mind off her recent loss. (Another possibility to expand your social circle is to perform a service, volunteer, administer a "contest" etc.)

Your financial planner and accountant should always be consulted when you are considering changes in your investment portfolio. Investments should not be bought or sold because of rumors in the neighborhood. Be leery of investment tips to buy "hot" stocks. Investments demand expertise and thoughtfulness if they are going to benefit you. Your accountant can help with any impact such a change could have on your income taxes.

Rely on your financial planner. He or she will develop a comprehensive financial plan for you, a plan which includes specific investment recommendations and options. Your financial advisor, if licensed, can also assist you in implementing your investment plan. The reality is, the investment choices that you will be confronted with are simply too complicated to try and sort out without a trusted advisor.

No credible planner would present the options to you and then leave them to you to bring to fruition. Your financial planner can be your partner in your financial well-being. By using a financial planner and an investment advisor, you stand to get the best of both worlds, particularly if your needs cannot be met by only one.

An Investment Plan

Your investment plan is a very important aspect of your overall financial plan. Savings as previously discussed, should never be included as investable dollars.

Always subtract savings from investable dollars. Because all investments carry some degree of risk — not to mention the fact that often investments demand long-term commitments to avoid penalties — your savings cannot be tied up in them.

Once you have determined how much you can safely invest — including IRAs and retirement plans — you can begin to plot out your investment plan.

"When I first sat down with an advisor," Harriet, another client of mine, shared, "it was as if she was speaking a foreign language. Fortunately, she was very patient explaining everything to me."

Your introduction to investments might be a confusing experience. This is just another reason why your advisor should be one that you trust and with whom you are comfortable. Check with family or friends on who they trust and with whom they are comfortable working with. If that doesn't turn up anyone, you can check with your accountant or lawyer. Make sure you choose someone who you are comfortable questioning. Remember, this is your money. There is no such thing as a "silly" question.

An income portfolio must, by nature, be more conservative and produce less volatility. Subsequently, it also produces less growth. For example, when you buy a fixed income investment like a US Treasury Bond, you are lending money to the securest and safest entity in the world. (Investment vehicles offered by the US government are the benchmark for the rest of the fixed income market.) Companies and countries that are trying to entice you to invest in their bonds (lend money to them in return for paying you interest and eventually returning your principal), all have to pay an interest rate to you that is higher then a US Treasury Bond.

If your late husband or you did a good job in setting up income streams now or in the future, then minimal risk needs to be taken. One of the concepts you need to understand is what we call the "permission slip" concept.

By setting up your assets so you can spend down principal, you can have more income during retirement without taking any unnecessary risk. Certain strategies help make this possible. For example, life insurance enables you to live better during retirement since it gave you a permission slip to spend principal and then eventually replace it with the life insurance proceeds. You may also choose to leave the insurance proceeds to charity if you have no heirs.

Inflation

Inflation is the true enemy of prudent investing. If a loaf of bread cost seven cents more and your investments have only earned you six cents then in spite of having "more money" your investments have lost ground in terms of buying power. They have not done their job.

Inflation erodes your purchasing power, making it more difficult to secure necessities, let alone luxuries.

When your husband was alive, his income tended to "keep pace" with inflation. That is, the likelihood was that his salary was adjusted yearly to remain ahead of inflation. However, now that you are relying more on fixed income generated from CDs and US Treasury Bonds, what will happen? (If possible, request that the income from your husband's old business have an inflation index to it.)

According to the Department of Labor, the average yearly rate of inflation over the past quarter century has been five percent. At that rate, $1,000 in the mattress is worth only half as much in fifteen years.

With inflation at the same rate, $100,000 loses $62,000 in purchasing power in just twenty years. What might seem like a significant amount of money when you first become a widow, may be whittled away to much, much less as time marches on.

One of the most important objectives of your widowhood is to assure sufficient income for your lifetime. You cannot allow yourself to get "caught short." Neglecting to account for the effect of inflation at any stage of your planning could result in exactly that unwelcome situation.

Your primary investment goal must be to stay ahead of inflation.

Systematic Savings and Withdrawals

One of the goals you should set for yourself is making your life easier. By this, I mean in the greater sense of setting up investments which will make your life financially secure as well as in the "lesser" sense of removing as many of the day-to-day hassles of life as possible.

Systematic savings and withdrawals is one small way to make life easier. Rather than receive your investment or Social Security checks in the mail and then have to physically take them to the bank, it is possible to arrange for direct deposit.

In addition to simplifying your life, direct deposit minimizes the risk of a check getting lost. Once all your income goes to a central account or location such as a money market account, then a monthly distribution program can be set up with your checking account.

Another advantage of this method is that your money is earning interest all the time, right to the point of spending it. Record keeping is also made easier by setting up such a program.

In addition to the pleasure of minimizing paperwork, a systematic savings program eliminates the need to be disciplined enough to save.

Annuities

Although annuities have received more than their share of "bad press," they are not necessarily bad. Your situation might warrant annuities. Remember, financial planning is a very individual process. There are no boilerplates, that is, one size does not fit all. What is good for you may not be good for someone else.

Some annuities create immediate income. Others do not. Those that do not will be able to create income at a future date, usually retirement. This income is either delayed or deferred income. (Remember, it is income tax deferred only when it's accumulating, not when you're receiving it.)

A deferred annuity takes two forms, variable and fixed. "Variable" means that the investment income will vary based on the performance of the underlying investment. "Fixed" means that the annuity will pay a guaranteed interest rate for a specified period of time. This guarantee is underwritten by an insurance company. (Make sure the insurance company is highly rated by at least two large independent rating agencies such as Moody's and A.M. Best.)

If you are in need of more income immediately, another possibility of an immediate annuity is to provide that higher income stream to you. Not only is the payment stream potentially higher compared to another fixed income vehicle such as a CD, but it is also guaranteed by the insurance company. (If any investment has a guaranteed portion it will also seem to pay a lower interest rate then some non-guaranteed investment vehicles.) In addition, since part of the income stream you receive back from an annuity is considered a return of capital, not all of the income received is subject to income taxes.

Please consult your own tax, legal or accounting professional before making any decision.

Summary - Chapter 14

1. Have your investment portfolio thoroughly reviewed.
2. By using a financial planner and an investment advisor, you stand to get the best of both worlds, particularly if your needs cannot be met by only one. Ask family, a friend, or an advisor who they would recommend.
3. There is no such thing as a "silly" question.

KEY WEBSITES:

Investment Planning;

www.mymoney.gov

Investment Questionnaire;

www.4TFG.com

Saving;

www.americasavesweek.org
www.saveandinvest.org

CHAPTER 15

Beware of Credit

"I try to avoid using my credit card except for certain purchases — and those I try to pay off as soon as the bill is due," my mother would always state with conviction.

My mother is on solid ground when she voices that sentiment. Avoid credit cards as much as possible. Credit card interest is very high, usually much more than you can earn and, in a double-whammy, is not tax deductible.

You can control spending. If you don't have the money in your checking account, you can't spend it. Credit cards are seductive because they allow you to spend more — sometimes much more — than you have. Stay within your budget or income level.

Remember, your goal is to have enough income to maintain your lifestyle for what will hopefully be a very long time.

Rule One: Don't Spend More than You Have!

Sounds simple, yes? However, judging by the difficulty so many people have with this simple rule, it is worth repeating. Don't spend more than you have! It is paramount to a good investment plan to remain within your asset and income limits.

Being wise and prudent cannot help but benefit your investment portfolio in the long run.

Summary — Chapter 15

1. Avoid using credit cards except for certain purposes.
2. Pay off credit card bills as soon as they are due.
3. Don't live above your means.

KEY WEBSITES:

Beware of credit "quick fixes";

www.thebeehive.org/money

Free credit reports;

www.credit.com

CHAPTER 16

Retirement Planning

"There are only two things in life you can't avoid..."
my mother would remind us.

Introduction

What could possibly sound easier than ending your working life? Leisure time. Financial freedom. Sleeping late in the morning... however, planning for your retirement so that you can enjoy all that leisure time can be very complicated. The government has devised regulations which can be confusing, even for the professional. It is to your benefit that these regulations be explained to you by someone knowledgeable in the field, a financial planner, tax attorney, investment professional, actuary (pension specialist), or an accountant.

What Makes Up Your Qualified Retirement Plans?

Individual Retirement Accounts (IRAs), Simplified Employee Pension (SEP), Keogh's, 401(k)s, 403(b)s, Pension and Profit Sharing plans all contribute to your "qualified retirement plans." Tax deferred, these plans will be subject to income taxes only when you withdraw and receive the money accruing in them.

Review a summary of your qualified retirement plans carefully so that you know your options.

Income tax will be due when you choose to withdraw the money or when you are obligated to withdraw the money. At the time of mandatory withdrawal, the minimum withdrawal is based on an Internal Revenue table and thetotal balance in all accounts. (You can split IRAs if you have more then one child or use a trust as the beneficiary. The rules using trusts as beneficiaries are complicated so make sure you seek competent advice before designating a beneficiary.)

Certain retirement monies cannot become a Rollover IRA. Defined Benefit Pension Plans have predetermined beneficiary options. As a result, there is no lump sum available for you to roll over into an IRA. You will receive the same monthly benefit or percentage of your husband's monthly benefit as stipulated in the Plan.

All interest, dividends and capital gains will remain tax deferred as long as they remain in the IRA. Investing in this account should be consistent with your overall investment objectives, including having taxable bonds in retirement accounts.

Have different exit strategies from retirement plans explained to you. For example, you can set up a "Charitable Remainder Trust" to coincide with a withdrawal from a retirement account. The income tax created by the withdrawal can be offset with the charitable income tax deduction from the "Charitable Remainder Trust".

Have your financial planner or accountant develop a schedule which will show you exactly which withdrawal program will minimize taxes and maximize what you and your heirs receive.

Summary - Chapter 16

1. Review a summary of your qualified retirement plans carefully so that you know your options.
2. Monies left in a qualified retirement plan are income tax deferred until they are withdrawn.
3. Have your financial planner develop a schedule which will show you how to minimize taxes (income and estate) and maximize benefits to you and your family.

KEY WEBSITES:

Retirement planning calculators;

www.yourretirementcalculation.com

CHAPTER 17

Estate Planning

My mother would always tell me to tell them to, "Take Care of Your Own Financial Future First!"

While this might seem obvious, it bears repeating — Secure your own financial future first and foremost. Before establishing an estate plan, your own needs must be met. You must be very comfortable with your income sources and with your ability to cover your expenses. Only then can you consider estate planning — and if you even need estate planning.

You should establish a balance between "saving for a rainy day" and enjoying each and every day of your life to the utmost. Your children's inheritance is important but not as important as your own enjoyment and well-being.

Durable Power of Attorney, Health Care Proxy and Living Will

While the Constitution makes very clear what happens if and when the President is incapacitated, you must do the same for yourself if you want to be sure to have your wishes observed in the event that you cannot make financial decisions for yourself. A "Power of Attorney" can help you accomplish this. All powers should be durable, that is the power is still valid in the event of a disability. If you have some apprehension giving someone such broad power, you can create a "springing power." A "springing" power of attorney only takes effect when you are unable to make such decisions, while a "durable" power of attorney goes into effect immediately after it is signed.

Your health proxy allows one of your relatives or trusted friends to make health care decisions for you if you are unable to make such decisions yourself.

Finally, depending on your personal and religious views regarding such things, you might want to consider a living will, which delineates your wishes regarding artificial life support should you become terminally ill.

Each of these documents can be prepared by yourself or an attorney. While it is possible to create these documents yourself using "boiler plates" available online, be aware of the common mistakes of an improper signature and a notary not included. An attorney's input will guarantee that the documents are legally binding and communicate exactly what you want them to communicate.

Should you decide to have such documents prepared, be sure to let your children or other close relative know where they are kept. You might even want your child to hold them in their possession.

Beneficiary Designations

Beneficiary designations are generally required for all IRAs, retirement plans, life insurance, and annuities.

Selecting your beneficiaries should be done in conjunction with the rest of your planning. If your estate is not exceptionally large and if your children or other beneficiaries are of age, then you should simply go ahead and name them formally as your beneficiaries.

For estate preservation planning, which I will discuss more completely below, you might find it preferable to take IRA withdrawals, pay any income taxes which are due, and then gift the monies out of your estate.

If your beneficiaries are minors, or in your view irresponsible, or you're worried about in-laws, you should consider a trust in your will and then making your estate or the trust your formal beneficiary.

Estate Taxes

The amount of your estate subject to taxes upon your death depends on the size and location of your estate. The Internal Revenue Service and your state government have estate tax tables to determine which tax bracket your estate is in if any. They are two separate and independent taxing authorities.

Everything that you own at your death is appraised at its "fair market value." Remember, your estate includes all your assets — home (including furnishings and personal items), bank accounts, brokerage accounts, retirement plans, business interests, life insurance proceeds, etc.

Life insurance can be removed from your estate if the owner is changed more than three years before your death to someone other then yourself. Typically the policy is transferred to an irrevocable trust, to your children or to charity. The details of such a transfer can be explained by one of your advisors.

In this context, perhaps the most important list you can make is one which lists instructions for your personal property as to who gets what and why. This list can serve as an emotional legacy that helps keep your family united rather than divided. (See List 7 in Chapter 6.)

Too many feuds and too much bitterness is engendered by misunderstandings about inheritance — of property both real and liquid.

Lists shouldn't be taken lightly. Even the lists stuck with a magnet to your refrigerator door. They clarify the situation. At the very least, that makes them a worthwhile time investment. A list is not a Will! Only a properly executed Will can be used in court to accomplish your wishes after you die. Major items should remain in your Will, but smaller, more personal belongings can be appropriately dealt with in a list.

No Will

Not having a clearly written legal Will is how "long lost" relatives may end up with a piece of your estate. It's also how extra costs, taxes, and delays are created.

Most importantly, it is also how children get "disinherited." If you remarry without a clear pre or post-nuptial agreement, or some other waiver signed by your new husband, your children can be left out in the cold. For example, without a pre-nuptial agreement in New York, a new husband is allowed one-third of your estate.

In most states, unless properly planned, husbands are not allowed to be disinherited. They are entitled by law to receive part of the estate. Should this happen, the amount of money your children receive at your death might go to your second husband's children from his previous marriage.

Your Will

Your executor/executrix is responsible for your estate when you die. His/her (even, their) main responsibility will be to select someone to probate and settle your estate in the state inwhich you are living when you die, making sure all debts are satisfied and all taxes paid. Your executor/executrix is also responsible to see to it that the terms of your Will are met.

Even if your estate is not so large to require estate taxes, you should still have a Will. Only through your Will can you determine which of your personal items (not those owned by your living trust or joint property with any of your children) will go to the person you want.

Make sure your Will contains something called a self-proving affidavit. A self-proving affidavit avoids an extra step by the surrogate court at your death. That is, locating the witnesses that signed your Will, wherever they may be located, to verify that they actually witnessed you signing your Will. If they are no longer alive, then a death certificate must be produced. As you can imagine, this can get rather complicated and cause some delays.

Accomplishing Your Intent with Your Assets

"The best intentions..."

Your Will should be reviewed regularly to make sure that it states clearly what you intend and that your intentions can be carried out. A client of mine drafted her Will to indicate that her two children were to inherit some property equally. She stated so emphatically in her Will. Unfortunately, the property was listed in joint name with her son, which took precedence over her Will, and so the daughter missed out.

Beneficiary designations of qualified retirement plans and life insurance need to be checked as well. If you have young children, the beneficiary should be your estate or a previously set up trust. The logic of this is to prevent your young children from inheriting their money outright when they reach legal age which, depending on the state in which you live, could be as young as eighteen.

If you name your estate as your beneficiary, then the assets will be controlled by your Will and they will go where you want them to go, rather than where your children want them to go. Remember, a young person who receives a substantial sum of money at a young age might have little incentive to finish school or go to work. That young child can also become vulnerable to unscrupulous people.

Of course, you can set up specific provisions in your Will that a trust be established and that the monies be reinvested until specific needs or occurrences come about, such as college graduation or attaining a certain age.

While such provisions might seem overly controlling at first glance, you will be doing your child a service in the long run. And, of course, you can include such language in your Will which will allow the trustee to invade principal as needed for the health, welfare, and maintenance of your child(ren).

If your intent is to guarantee funds for a child with special needs, you might consider a life insurance policy for that purpose. This life insurance will be setup in an irrevocable trust, sometimes referred to as a Crummey Trust, named after a famous court case, which established the basis for such an insurance trust.

A trust called a special needs trust can also be prepared by an attorney whereby your child can still qualify for Federal or state assistance from Social Security or Medicaid.

Choosing a Residency

It sounds simple but the best place to live is where you're going to be happy. If that's nearer to your children or closer to the ocean or someplace where it's always, always warm, then that's where you should live.

One of my clients sold her house after her husband died. She went to another state to live closer to her son and daughter. Both of whom were in their late thirties and hadn't lived near their mother since leaving for college. The move proved to be a boon to their relationships. My client was an "ever-present" grandparent and friend to her son and daughter.

An added benefit to moving was leaving a house which held so many memories that were increasingly difficult for her to deal with. The house also promised to be a financial drain. Old houses and apartments demand significant maintenance and repair.

Florida and Nevada are well known "retirement" states. They have great climates, except in the summer, and a lower cost of living than states in the Northeast. Not only do certain states cost less to live, they cost less to die.

While that may not be a primary consideration in your choice of where to live, if you want to save estate taxes for your children, consider a state with little or no estate taxes.

Living Trusts (Revocable)

I was in an attorney's office with some of my clients when the attorney asked, "Do you know why living trusts are so popular in Florida?"

No one answered although the answer seemed obvious

when he gave it. "Because so many people die there, the courts get very backed up."

Florida or not, after many meetings with attorneys, I have come to the conclusion that if you own a significant number of assets, a living trust is a wonderful option to consider.

The living trust, once all your assets are transferred into it, becomes a vehicle through which you can control your assets.

As trustee, you receive all income, make all buying and selling decisions, and determine the ultimate disposition or continuity of the trust at your death. You also determine provisions should you become incapacitated.

The goal is always control. Depending on your circumstances, a living trust might afford you the greatest number of options and the greatest degree of control.

Lifetime Gifting

I remember sitting with a prospective client, a gentleman in his middle eighties. When discussing his family, he told me about his son, a man in his fifties, who, according to the father, "didn't know the value of a buck."

My reaction was straightforward. If he didn't know the value of a buck by his stage in life, chances were he was never going to learn. I counseled my prospective client that he might as well let his son benefit from his money rather than force him to wait until he died.

"I don't see any benefit to you or your son by waiting." While your own children might very well "know the value of a buck," if you have extra money and want to minimize the amount of money going for estate taxes, it makes sense to make whatever gifts are permissible under current gift and estate tax laws.

Currently, the IRS allows annual gifts to any relative, friend or person. Gift tax rules should be checked at your state level to make sure that the same amount applies. In addition, a grandparent can pay unlimited amounts directly for medical or educational bills of the donee because they are not considered gifts for gift tax purposes. (The funds should be paid to the provider of medical services or the educational institution, not to the donee.)

Gifts can be in the form of cash or other assets. Again, consult with your advisor to determine which asset is the best one to gift. Remember, once you gift it, the asset is gone. In matters of taxation, there are no "give backs."

Have your advisor prepare a "cash flow model," one which clearly shows the impact that your gifts may have on your lifestyle, before starting a gifting program. Then, if you can afford to make the gifts, by all means, do it.

If you find yourself uncomfortable gifting money to your children outright, give some thought to the various education tax incentives which are available for qualified tuition and related expenses (i.e., tuition and fees, but not room and board or books). Your accountant or financial advisor will explain to you what options, if any, are available if you qualify.

Gifts to children or grandchildren can also go directly into custodian accounts. These accounts are relatively easy to establish if you have the child's social security number. Custodian accounts give the child the legal right under state law, to receive the money at a specified age. The state law is derived from one of two legal forms, referred to as either Uniform Gifts to Minors Act (UGMA) or the Uniform Transfers to Minors Act (UTMA). Depending on the child's age, it may be subject to income tax at the child's level or at the parent's level. If you're the custodian, the money is still in your estate, so consider another custodian other then yourself.

Another way to get money to a child, is by using an "in trust for" account designation at a bank, called a Totten Trust. No actual gift is made with this account since the assets are still in your name. The only time the child becomes owner of the account is when you die and they inherit it. Tax waivers may be required before the money can be released to the child or grandchild, depending on the amount in the account. Consider instead, setting up an educational trust through an attorney, which would potentially delay the receipt of the money by the child until they graduate from college.

My mother's view is that she'd rather see her children and grandchildren enjoying the money while she's still alive. As a personal note, I appreciate my mother's perspective profoundly. However, I recognize that not everyone shares my mother's view.

One of the most advantageous uses of gifts, particularly if your estate will eventually be subject to estate taxes, is to have your child(ren) or a trust, purchase a life insurance policy on your life. This use of gifts to purchase life insurance can maximize a limited amount of funds that you have to give away. You can also purchase the life insurance without a trust incase you ever need access to the cash value.

Life insurance is an excellent source of instant cash for your family at the exact time that they need it — when income taxes, estate taxes or administrative costs are due.

If your children are not responsible or if divorce and

lawsuits are a possibility then an irrevocable trust with the children as trustees should be used. The trustee(s) become(s) the owner(s) and beneficiary(ies) of the life insurance policy and are governed by the trust document. The concept is the same as using the children directly, except that in this instance, the trustee is the recipient of the gift and then pays the insurance company. The trust can protect the insurance proceeds from divorce, lawsuits, and estate taxes if applicable.

If such a trust is established, it becomes its own separate tax-paying entity, with its own checking account and a tax identification number from the IRS. A knowledgeable attorney should be consulted to set up the trust.

A financial planner who specializes in life insurance and estate planning is your best contact for purchasing a policy. Most large financial institutions have in-house experts in this area. Establish a relationship with an expert that you are comfortable with, someone with whom you can establish a long-term relationship.

I cannot tell you how many widows I've spoken with who tell me that their husbands didn't "believe in life insurance." My reaction varies depending on the situation, but generally speaking, I explain that life insurance is a valuable financial tool which creates a number of options.

If you have young children or children who are still establishing themselves, you should have an analysis done to determine what shortages they would have should you die tomorrow.

Trustee's Role

The role of the trustee is really quite simple. He or she

is responsible to carry out the provisions of whatever trust you set up now or in your Will. For performing this role, the trustee is entitled to a well-earned fee — unless this has been waived. Well-earned because the trustee acts in a caretaker capacity, a fiduciary capacity, which includes the responsibility of making sure all tax forms are filed in a timely manner and that any and all available monies are properly invested.

If the trust is set up for your children and they are also named as trustees, then trying to limit the principal or income they can receive — unless specifically spelled out — will not work. By the same token, putting trustees in place who are located in other states, or who will be insensitive to the needs of the trust beneficiaries, will not work either.

This is one area where the wrong choice can have serious and damaging consequences. Choosing a trustee is a very important decision.

Getting an Estate Plan Done

If you think that you might require an estate plan, speak to an estate planner. An estate planner can take the title of attorney, financial planner, CPA, life insurance agent, or even a private banker, such as a trust officer.

Find someone who you are comfortable with and who you can afford. The important thing is to find someone you like and trust and can get the job done.

Summary — Chapter 17

1. Your children's inheritance is important, but not as important as your own enjoyment and well-being.
2. Have an attorney prepare a durable power of attorney and a health proxy for you.
3. Check your beneficiary designations on all retirement accounts, annuities, and life insurance policies.
4. Make sure your Will is current and has a self-proving affidavit attached.
5. If you are insurable, consider a permanent life insurance policy to give you options in the future.
6. Consider lifetime gifts only after a cash flow projection (comparing your income to your expense) has been done.

KEY WEBSITES:

General Estate Planning info;

www.4tfg.com

CHAPTER 18

Importance of Financial Planning

"Believe it or not, keeping track of the finances does become easier," my mother would proudly state.

"Fail to Plan, Plan to Fail"

The need for financial planning has become more and more important. I believe the main reason for this is that financial choices have become more complicated. There are more mutual funds, insurances, and advisors to choose from then ever before. Someone is touting something that is better then the next. The media shows you this every day.

However, the key, before any product or choice is made, is to have a plan. Would you go on a long trip where you've never been before without some sort of map or tour guide?

Of course not. Nor should you plan for your financial future without a plan. Your plan is a road map to get you where you want to go. The road is filled with many detours and pot holes. You need to do your best to get to your destination with the least amount of hassle and inconvenience.

In financial planning, where you want to go is vital information in deciding how to get there.

Think With Your Head and Not With Your Heart

Certain issues previously mentioned are not all that simple to implement. Sometimes things are easier said then done. You want to realize that particular issues are going to touch buttons. Expect it and do your best in dealing with the different emotions as they arise.

The last section to follow is potentially one of the more difficult issues in which your emotions can get in your way. This is why rational thinking needs to prevail.

Lending Money to Your Children

Clearly, there are aspects to this discussion which go far beyond the appropriate realm of financial advice. The decisions of money lending to members of your family may have been affected by the death of your husband. You alone have to determine whether or not to lend money to your children, whereas before you would have been able to discuss it with your husband.

In spite of the successful relationship I enjoy with my mother, we have our differences with reference to money. When I asked her if I could borrow a large sum of money, she hesitated for fear of losing her income. However, after much thought, she did give me the loan.

Given my own experience, I suggest that when your child comes to you for money — and has an objectively valid reason and need — you should give or lend your child the money. If you can afford it and if the money is given in the right way and for the right purpose, everyone benefits.

Gifts and loans are an appropriate and easily managed financial matter. Your accountant, lawyer, or financial advisor can guide you in how best to accomplish the exchange of money, and what interest rate you should charge for a loan.

Again, if you are able and if the request is valid, I would urge you to honor it. If you do not, there is likely to be damaging emotional consequences. As an accountant and investment advisor representative offering investment advisory services through 4Thought Financial Group Inc. (4TFG). (Securities offered through American Portfolios Financial Services Inc. (APFS) member of FINRA/SIPC. APFS is not affiliated with 4TFG), I know very well the worth of money. As a son, husband and father, I also know the value of family.

Your sense of well-being is likely derived from the love and support of your family as well as financial security. It is rarely worth the cost to family relationships to deny a loan or gift. I always ask my clients what the children will do with some of the personal assets at their death. My common answer is that the children will have a dumpster parked in the driveway and cart everything away. Some of the items that you might put such credence in, your children are only going to discard, so it's certainly not worth haggling over while you are alive.

Remember, ultimately all our considerations have to do with quality of life — your life. Your financial planning should be designed to ensure a comfort level for you and your emotional security.

Keep your family together as best you can. Too many families are spread out over vast geographical areas. Whenever possible, it is best to minimize the emotional space between family members.

The best investment I can recommend is to maintain the health and growth of family ties.

Summary — Chapter 18

1. "Fail to plan, plan to fail." Do not let it happen to you.
2. Do your best with the emotions as they arise.
3. Hold on to those family ties.

Afterword

I sincerely hope that this book will help you to surmount the loss of your life partner and best friend. He would want you to enjoy the best quality of life you can. This would have made him very happy to know that you were able to do so.

M.E.L.

NOTES

NOTES

NOTES

Made in United States
Troutdale, OR
02/16/2024

17737266R00086